QUICK MEDICAL TERMINOLOGY

Genevieve Love Smith

formerly, Coordinator of Programming
Point Park College
Pittsburgh, Pennsylvania

Phyllis E. Davis

formerly, Dean of the College
Point Park College
Pittsburgh, Pennsylvania

in consultation with
Shirley E. Soltesz, R.N., B.S.

Instructional Technologist

JOHN WILEY & SONS
New York • Chichester • Brisbane • Toronto • Singapore

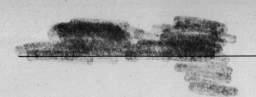

Library of Congress Catalog Card Number: 72-188144

ISBN 0-471-80198-4

Printed in the United States of America.

20 19 18

To the Reader

QUICK MEDICAL TERMINOLOGY teaches a system for building
thousands of medical terms. This self-teaching book is designed for
anyone who wishes to learn medical vocabulary, either because they
work in medicine or in a medically related field, or because of personal
interest. No special background is required, other than a high school
education or the equivalent. (Knowledge of anatomy might be helpful,
but is not necessary; illustrations provide some orientation to anatomical relationships.)

Because you will teach yourself, you will learn at your own pace.
Throughout the program you will actively participate--identifying word
parts, building new words, pronouncing them, practicing them. "The
Word-Building System"provides an introduction; the rest of the program,
divided into ten units, teaches you to apply the system, using new word
parts to form a constantly expanding medical vocabulary. You will
learn best if you complete a unit at one sitting, rather than stopping in
the middle.

Each unit is divided into numbered frames; each frame will provide
some information and will ask you a question. As soon as you have
written out your answer, you should check it against the answer given
in the left-hand column, to see whether or not you have mastered the
material. If your answer does not match the one given, be sure you
understand why not before you go on; if you have misspelled a word,
write out the correct answer. (Many people find it helpful to use a folded
piece of paper to cover the answers until they have completed a frame.)

Usually the answer to a frame will consist of just one word; often
diagonals are used to separate the word parts (_____/___/_____). If the
question calls for more than one word, there will be one asterisk at the
beginning of the answer blank (*_____). If you see two asterisks (**_____),
you are to use your own words in answering the question.

In the left-hand column, you will find not only the correct answers,
but often a guide to the pronunciation of a word. The program will be
most effective and enjoyable if you pronounce aloud each new word as

you form it. Later in the program when you are more familiar with medical terms, this guide is not given as often. However, you should always pronounce any new word you have formed before you go on to the next frame; if you are unsure about the pronunciation, check your dictionary. At the end of each chapter is a selected list of words introduced in that chapter; pronounce them aloud before proceeding.*

At the back of the book are review sheets for each chapter, which you can use at any time, as often as you wish. They are particularly useful before taking a test or if some time has elapsed between units. At the end of each chapter is a self-test with answers given on the following page. If you have more than six incorrect answers, either study the review sheets or go through the unit again before starting a new unit. As always, if your answer does not agree with the one given, be sure you understand why before you go on.

The glossary of word parts, also at the back of the book, lists where each word part was introduced in the program. And if you wish to expand your medical vocabulary still more, you may use the list of additional word parts with a medical dictionary.

Two final tests are also provided. You may wish to take one before starting the book and the other after finishing, to see how much you have actually learned. If so, turn to page 235. Otherwise go on to the Objectives of the Program and the Word-Building System.

G. L. S.
P. E. D.
S. E. S.

May 1972

*A 60-minute optional pronunciation cassette is now available to accompany this Guide. The tape cassette costs $8.95 (price subject to change without notice). The word parts at the beginning and the word list at the end of each chapter are pronounced, and the student can compare his pronunciation with that on the tape. To order the cassette or to obtain further information, send in the green card at the back of this book.
**A set of crossword puzzles specially designed for reviewing medical terminology have been created by Deanna Hardin, R.N., Coordinator of Inservice Education at Medical City Dallas Hospital and Instructor at El Centro College, Dallas, Texas. These puzzles are available without charge from the publisher. To order the Medical Terminology Crossword Puzzles, write to:

Editor, Self-Teaching Guides
John Wiley & Sons, Inc.
605 Third Avenue
New York, N.Y. 10016

Contents

Objectives of the Program

When you have finished QUICK MEDICAL TERMINOLOGY, you will have formed over 500 medical terms using the word-building system, combining Greek and Latin prefixes, suffixes, word roots, and combining forms. You should then be able to:

1. recognize and understand these word parts in your daily use of medical terminology

2. build appropriate medical terms from the word parts you have learned, given the meaning of a word

3. identify new word parts in other medical terms and, having learned their meanings, to be able to use these new word parts to both build and understand further medical terms, following this word-building system.

The Word-Building System

QUICK MEDICAL TERMINOLOGY teaches a system of word building. It has exceptions, of course, but once you have learned the system you will be able to build thousands of words. Medicine has a large vocabulary, but you can learn much of it by following the system and putting words together from their parts.

1
All words have a word root. This is the foundation of a word. The foundation of trans/port, ex/port, im/port, and sup/port is the word root

port

_____.

2
Suf/fix, pre/fix, af/fix, and fix/ation have fix

word root

as their *_____.

3
What is the word root in tonsill/itis, tonsill/

tonsill

ectomy, and tonsill/ar? _____.

4
Compound words are formed when two (or more) word roots are used to build the word. Even in ordinary English, compound words are formed

word roots

from two or more *_____.

5

Sometimes the two word roots are words.
They still form a compound word. Is short/

Yes.
It is formed from
two words: short
and hand

hand a compound word? _____. Explain

your answer. ** _____

_____.

6

Form a compound word, using the words under

underage

and age: _____.

7

Form a compound word from the word roots

chickenpox

chicken and pox: _____.

8

A combination of two or more words or two or
more word roots means that the word formed is

compound word

a * _____.

9

A combining form is word root plus a vowel.
In the word therm/o/meter, the combining form

therm/o

is _____/____.

10

In the word speed/o/meter, speed/o is the

combining form

* _____.

11

In the compound words micr/o/scope, micr/o/

micr

film, and micr/o/be, the word root is _____;

micr/o

the combining form is _____/____.

12

Compound words can also be formed from a combining form of the word root and a whole word. In the word therm/o/meter, the com-

therm/o

bining form is _____/____ ; the whole

meter

word is _____ .

13

In each of the following compound words, circle the whole word. Underline just the word root:

micr/o/film

micr/o/film

hydr/o/meter

hydr/o/meter

14

In medical terminology, compound words are usually built from a combining form, a word root, and an ending. In the word micr/o/scop/ ic,

micr/o

the combining form is _____/____ ;

scop

the word root is _____ ;

ic

the ending is _____ .

15

Build a word from
the combining form   electr/o,
the word root   stat,
the ending   ic.

electr/o/stat/ic

_____/____ /_____/____ .

16

In the word electr/o/metr/ic,

combining form

electr/o is the *_____ ;

word root

metr is the *_____ ;

ending

ic is the _____ .

17

The ending that follows a word root is a suffix.
In the words plant/er, plant/ed, plant/ing, the

er, ed, ing   suffixes are _____, _____, _____.

18

You can change the meaning of a word by adding
a suffix. The suffix er means one who. The
word root port means to carry. When you add
the suffix er (port/er), the word means

one who carries   ** _____.

19

Able changes the meaning of read in the word

suffix   read/able; able is a _____.

20

A prefix is a word part that goes before a word,
or some form of a word, and changes its meaning. In the words im/plant, sup/plant, and

im, sup,   trans/plant, the prefixes are _____, _____,

trans   _____.

21

In the word dis/please, dis comes before and
changes the meaning of please; dis is a

prefix   _____.

22

Before studying more, review what you have
learned. The foundation of a word is called the

word root   * _____.

23

A word that is placed before a word to change

prefix   its meaning is a _____.

24

A word part that follows a word root is a

suffix   _____.

25

When a vowel is added to a word root, the word

part that results is called the * _____

combining form   _____.

26

When some form of two or more word roots is
combined to form a word, that word is called a

compound word   *_____.

Unit 1

In Unit 1 you will make 24 new words by using the following word root-combining forms and suffixes:

acr/o (extremities)
cardi/o (heart)
cyan/o (blue)
cyt/o (cell)
dermat/o, derm/o (skin)
duoden/o (duodenum)

electr/o (electrical)
gastr/o (stomach)
gram/o (record)
leuk/o (white)
megal/o (enlarged)

-al (adjective ending)
-algia (pain)
-ectomy (excision of)
-itis (inflammation of)
-ologist (one who studies, a
  specialist)

-ology (study of)
-osis (condition of)
-ostomy (forming a new opening)
-otomy (incision into)
-tome (instrument that cuts)
-um, -y, -a, -ia (noun endings)

	1 Acr/o is used to build words that refer to the extremities. To refer to extremities, physi-
acr/o or acr	cians use words containing _____/___.
	2 Acr/o is found in words concerning the extremities, which in the human body are the arms and legs. To build words about the arms, use
acr/o	_____/___.
	3
acr/o	To build words about the legs, use _____/___.

4

Acr/o any place in a word should make you think of the extremities. When you read a word containing acr or acr/o, you think of

extremities

_____.

5

The words acr/o/megaly (acromegaly), acr/o/cyan/osis (acrocyanosis), and acr/o/dermat/itis (acrodermatitis) all refer to the

extremities

_____.

6

Megal/o means enlarged. Megal/o can also mean large. A word containing megal/o will

large, big, or
   enlarged

mean that something is _____.

7

Acr/o/megal/y (acromegaly) means that the

large, big, or
   enlarged

extremities are _____.

8

Acr/o/megal/y means enlargement of the extremities. The word that means a person has

acr/o/megal/y
acromegaly
ak ro meg' a li

enlarged hands is _____ / / / .

9

Occasionally you see a person with very large hands, feet, nose, and chin. His skin also has a coarse texture. He probably has

acromegaly

_____.

10

Dermat/o refers to the skin. A dermat/o/logist (dermatologist) is a specialist in a field of medicine. He specializes in diseases of the

skin

_____.

acr/o/dermat/itis
acrodermatitis
ak ro der ma ti' tis

11
Acr/o/dermat/itis (acrodermatitis) is a word
that means inflammation of the skin of the extremities. A person with red, inflamed hands

has _____ / / _____ / _____ .

12
A simpler way to say that a patient is suffering
from an inflammation of the hands, lower arms,
feet, and legs is to say that he has

acrodermatitis

_____ .

13
Remembering that the word acrodermatitis
means inflammation of the skin of the extremities, draw a conclusion; itis is a suffix that

inflammation   — means _____ .

14
Cyan/o is used in words to mean blue or blueness. Acr/o/cyan/osis means blueness of the
extremities. The part of the word that tells

cyan or cyan/o   you that the color blue is involved is _____ / ___ .

15
The suffix osis makes a word a noun and means
condition. To describe a condition of blueness

osis   of the extremities, use the suffix _____ .

noun   Acrocyanosis is a _____ (noun/verb).

acr/o/cyan/osis
acrocyanosis
ak ro si a no' sis

16
Acrocyanosis, or blueness of the extremities,
is usually related to the amount of oxygen get-
ting to the hands and feet. When the heart
doesn't pump enough blood containing oxygen,

the patient exhibits _____ / / _____ / ___ .

17

When the lungs cannot get enough oxygen into
the blood because of asthma, blueness of the
extremities may result. This is another cause

acrocyanosis

of _____.

18

blueness of the
  extremities

Acrocyanosis means ** _____

_____.

19

Dermat/osis means any skin condition. This
word denotes an abnormal skin condition. The

osis

suffix that means condition is _____.

20

cyan/osis
cyanosis
si an o' sis

Osis is a suffix, forms a noun, and means a
condition. Build a word that means a condition

of blueness. _____/_____.

21

dermat/osis
dermatosis
der mat o' sis

Build a word that means condition of the skin.

_____/_____.

22

The Greek work <u>tomos</u> means a piece cut off.
From this word we have many combining forms
that refer to cutting: ec/tom/y (cut out),
o/tom/y (cut into), tome (an instrument that
cuts). A dermatome is an instrument that cuts

skin

_____.

23

dermat/ome
dermatome
der' ma tōm

A dermatome is an instrument. When a physician wants a thin slice of a patient's skin for a

skin graft, he will ask for a _____/____.

24
Derm/o is another combining form for words referring to the skin. Cyan/o/derm/a

(cyanoderma) means ** _____

_____ .

a bluish discolor-
ation of the skin

25
Cyanoderma sometimes occurs when children swim too long in cold water. If a person has a bluish discoloration of the skin for any reason,

he suffers from _____ / / ____ / .

cyan/o/derm/a
cyanoderma
si an o der' ma

26
Leuk/o means white or abnormally white. In the compound word leuk/o/derm/a, the part

that means white is _____ .

leuk or leuk/o

27
Leuk/o/derm/a means ** _____

_____ .

white skin, or
abnormally
white skin

28
Some people have much less color in their skin than is normal. Their skin is white. They

have _____ / / ____ / .

leuk/o/derm/a
leukoderma
lu ko der' ma

29
Cyt/o refers to cells. Cytology is the study of cells. The part of cyt/o/logy that means cells

is _____ / .

cyt/o

30
There are several kinds of cells in blood. One kind is the leuk/o/cyte. A leukocyte is a

_____ blood _____ .

white blood cell

31

There are several different kinds of white blood cells in the blood. When a physician wants to know how many there are of all kinds, he will

leuk/o/cyt/e
leukocyte
lu' ko sīt

ask for a _____/___/_____ count.

32

You have heard of leuk/em/ia, popularly called "blood cancer"; ia is a noun ending and em stems from a Greek work meaning blood. A noun meaning literally "white blood" is

leuk/em/ia
leukemia
lu ke' mi a

_____/___/___.

33

In the word acr/o/megal/y, the combining form

acr/o

for extremities is _____/___ and the word

megal

root for big or large is _____.

34

large heart or
  enlargement of
  the heart

Cardi/o is the combining form for words about the heart. Megal/o/cardi/a is a noun that

means ** _____.

Esophagus

Heart

Liver

Gallbladder

Stomach

35
Megalocardia refers to heart muscle. When any muscle exercises, it gets larger. If the heart muscle has to overexericse,

megal/o/cardi/a
megalocardia
meg a lo kar' dia

_____ / / _____ / ___ will probably occur.

36
Inadequate oxygen supply causes the heart muscle to beat more often. An inadequate amount of oxygen can also lead to

megalocardia

_____.

37
Try this one. Gastr is the word root for stomach; ia is a noun ending. When the stomach enlarges so that it crowds other organs, an undesirable condition exists known as

megal/o/gastr/ia
megalogastria
meg a lo gas' tri a

_____ / / _____ / ___.

38
large heart or
  enlargement of
  the heart

Megalocardia means ** _____

_____.

39
Cardi/o is used in building words that refer to the heart. Card/itis means ** _____

inflammation of
  the heart

_____.

40
The combining forms logy and logist are suffixes you will use for convenience.
logos   - Greek for study,
log/y   - noun, study of,
log/ist - noun, one who studies.
A cardi/o/logist is a specialist in the study of

heart

diseases of the _____.

41

cardi/o/logist
cardiologist
kar di ol' o gist

A cardiologist diagnoses heart disease. The specialist who determines that a heart is deformed is a _____ / / _____.

42

cardiologist

A physician who reads electr/o/cardi/o/grams (records of electrical impulses given off by the heart) is also a _____.

43

a record of electrical waves given off by the heart (or equivalent)

Give the meaning of electr/o/cardi/o/gram. (Gram/o is a combining form that means record.) ** _____

_____.

44

electr/o/cardi/o/
    gram
electrocardiogram
e lek tro kar' di o
    gram

The electr/o/cardi/o/gram is a record obtained by electr/o/cardi/o/graph/y. A technician can learn electrocardiography, but it takes a cardiologist to read the

_____ / / _____ / / ____.

45

A physician can take a chart that looks like this,

and learn something about a person's heart. He

cardiologist

is a _____ and is read-

electrocardiogram

ing an _____.

46

cardi/algia
cardialgia
kar di al' ji a

The suffix algia means pain. Form a word that means heart pain. (Since algia is a suffix, you will use the word root for heart rather than the combining form.) _____ / _____.

47

When a patient complains of pain in the heart,
his symptom is known medically as

cardialgia

_____.

48

pain in the
  stomach

Gastralgia means ** _____

_____.   The suffix for pain

algia

is _____.

49

Gastr/ectomy means excision (removal) of all
or part of the stomach. Gastr/o is the combin-

stomach

ing form for _____. Ectomy is a
combining form that you may use as a suffix.

excision or
  removal

Ectomy means _____.

50

gastr/ectomy
gastrectomy
gas trek' to mi

A gastr/ectomy is a surgical procedure. When
a stomach ulcer has perforated, a partial

_____/_____ may be indicated.

51

Cancer of the stomach will result in a

gastrectomy

_____.

52

gastr/itis
gastritis
gas tri' tis

Form a word that means inflammation of the

stomach. _____/_____.

53

duoden/um
duodenum
du o dē' num

The duoden/um is the part of the small intestine
that connects with the stomach. Duoden/o is a
word root-combining form that refers to the

_____/____.

54

forming an opening
  between the
  stomach and
  duodenum

The combining form os/tom/y can be used as a suffix to mean forming an opening. Gastr/o/duoden/ostomy means ** _____

_____.

55

gastr/o/duoden/
  ostomy
gastroduodenostomy
gas tro du o den os'
  to mi

A surgeon who removes the natural connection between the duodenum and stomach and then forms a new connection is doing a

_____ / ____ / _____ / _____.

56

gastroduodenostomy

A gastroduodenostomy is a surgical procedure. When the pyloric sphincter, a valve that controls the amount of food going from the stomach to the duodenum, no longer functions, a

_____

may be done.

57

duodenum

The combining form o/tom/y means incision into. A duo/den/otomy is an incision into the

_____.

58

otomy

duoden/otomy
duodenotomy
du o den ot' o me

The suffix for incision into is _____.

Any time a surgeon has made an incision into the duodenum it is a _____ / _____.

59

duodenotomy

If a growth must be removed from the inner wall of the duodenum, a _____
is done.

itis

60
The suffix for inflammation is _____.

duoden/itis
duodenitis
du o den i' tis

The word inflammation of the duodenum is

_____/_____.

61
Duoden/al is an adjective; al is an adjectival ending meaning pertaining to (whatever the adjective modifies).   One adjectival ending is

al

_____.

62
In the sentence "Duodenal carcinoma was present," the adjective meaning pertaining to the

duoden/al
duodenal
du o de' nal

duodenum is _____/____.

63
The suffix ostomy means making a new opening. The word to form a new opening into the duo-

duoden/ostomy
duodenostomy
du o den os' to me

denum is _____/_____.

64
Here's one for you to figure out.   A duodenostomy can be formed in more than one manner. If it is formed with the stomach, it is called a

gastroduodenostomy

_____.

65
The suffix for forming a new opening is

ostomy

_____.

Use the material in the following chart to help work the next four frames.

WORDS ARE FORMED BY

I. Word root + suffix
   A. dermat/itis
   B. cyan/osis
   C. duoden/al
II. Combining form + word root + suffix
    (a suffix can be a word itself)
    A. acr/o/cyan/osis
    B. leuk/o/cyte
    C. megal/o/gastr/ia
III. Any number of combining forms + word root
     + suffix
    A. leuk/o/cyt/o/lys/is
    B. electr/o/cardi/o/graph/y

66
Form a word without even knowing its meaning.
Use what is needed from encephal/o + itis:

encephal/itis

_____/_____.

67
Use what is needed from   encephal/o
                          malac/o
                          ia

encephal/o/
 malac/ia

_____/ /_____/___.

68
Use what is needed from   encephal/o
                          mening/o
                          itis

encephal/o/
 mening/itis

_____/ /_____/___.

69
Use what is needed from encephal/o
                            myel/o
                            path/o
                            y

encephal/o/myel/
  o/path/y   _____ / / _____ / / ____ / __.

   While working through Unit 1, you formed the following 24 new medical terms. Read them one at a time and pronounce each aloud.

acrocyanosis	dermatome	gastrectomy
acrodermatitis	dermatosis	gastritis
acromegaly	duodenal	gastroduodenostomy
cardialgia	duodenitis	leukemia
carditis	duodenostomy	leukocyte
cardiologist	duodenotomy	leukoderma
cyanoderma	electrocardiogram	megalocardia
cyanosis	gastralgia	megalogastria

Before going on to Unit 2, take the Unit 1 Self-Test.

UNIT 1   SELF-TEST

PART 1

From the list on the right select the correct meaning for each of the
following terms. Write the letter in the space provided.

_____ 1. Megalocardia

_____ 2. Duodenostomy

_____ 3. Dermatologist

_____ 4. Gastritis

_____ 5. Electrocardiography

_____ 6. Gastralgia

_____ 7. Cardiologist

_____ 8. Acrocyanosis

a. A specialist in a field of skin
diseases

b. A condition of blueness of the
extremities

c. Enlargement of the heart

d. Forming a new opening in the
duodenum

e. A physician who specializes in
the study of the heart

f. Pain in the stomach

g. Inflammation of the stomach

h. Study of recordings of electrical
waves of the heart

PART 2

Write a medical term for each of the following:

1. A bluish discoloration of the skin   _____

2. A white blood cell   _____

3. Large or enlarged stomach   _____

4. A disease of too many white
cells in the blood   _____

5. Excision or removal of the
stomach   _____

6. Pertaining to the duodenum   _____

7. Heart pain   _____

ANSWERS

Part 1   Part 2

1. c   1. Cyanoderma
2. d   2. Leukocyte (also leukocytosis)
3. a   3. Megalogastria
4. g   4. Leukemia
5. h   5. Gastrectomy
6. f   6. Duodenal
7. e   7. Cardialgia
8. b

Unit 2

In Unit 2 you will put together at least 30 new words, using the following word root-combining forms, prefixes, and suffixes.

aden/o (gland)
arthr/o (joint)
carcin/o (malignancy)
cele/o, o/cele (hernia)
cephal/o (head)
chondr/o (cartilage)
cost/o (ribs)
dent/o (tooth)

emes/is (vomiting)
laryng/o (larynx)
lip/o (fat)
malac/o (soft)
oste/o (bone)
plast/o (repair)
troph/o (development)

en- (in, inside)
hyper- (over)
hypo- (under)
inter- (between)

-ia, -ic (pertaining to)
-oid (resembling)
-oma (tumor)

1
A prefix goes before a word to change its meaning. In the words hyper/trophy, hyper/emia, and hyper/emesis, the meaning of trophy, emia, and emesis is changed by hyper; hyper is a

prefix _____ that means above or more than normal.

2
Hyper/thyroid/ism means overactivity of the thyroid gland. The prefix that means the thyroid gland is secreting more than normal is

hyper _____.

hyper/emesis
hyperemesis
hi per em' e sis

3
Emesis is a word that means vomiting.   A word that means excessive vomiting is

_____ / _____ .

hyperemesis

4
Gallbladder attacks can cause excessive vomiting.   This, too, is called _____ .

hyper/trophy
hypertrophy
hi per' tro fi

5
Hyper/trophy means overdevelopment; troph/o comes from the Greek word for nourishment. Note the connection between nourishment and development.   Overdevelopment is called

_____ / _____ .

hypertrophy

6
Muscles also can overdevelop or

_____ .

hypertrophy

7
Many organs can overdevelop.   If the heart overdevelops, the condition is

_____ of the heart.

hypo

8
The prefix hypo is just the opposite of hyper. The prefix for under or less than normal is

_____ .

skin

skin

9
Derm/o refers to the _____ .   The suffix ic makes the word an adjective.   Hypo/derm/ic is an adjective that means under the _____ .

10

A hypodermic needle is short because it goes just under the skin. A shot that can be given superficially is administered with a

hypo/der/mic
hypodermic
hi po der' mic

_____/_____/_____ needle.

11

Aden/o is used in words that refer to glands. Build a word that means inflammation of a gland (word root + suffix rule):.

aden/itis
adenitis
ad en i' tis

_____/_____.

12

Since ectomy means excision or removal of, the word for removal of a gland is

aden/ectomy
adenectomy
ad en ek' to mi

_____/_____.

13

If a gland is tumorous, part or all of it may be excised. This operation is an

adenectomy

_____.

14

The suffix for tumor is oma. Form a word that means tumor of a gland:

aden/oma
adenoma
ad en o' ma

_____/_____.

15

Try this. Sometimes the thyroid gland develops a tumor. A patient's history might read, "... because of the presence of a thyroid adenoma, thyroidectomy is indicated." What is a thyroid/

removal, or
  excision, of the
  thyroid gland

ectomy? ** _____

_____.

16

tumor

fat

An adenoma is a glandular tumor; oma is the
suffix for _____. A lip/oma is a tumor
containing fat. Lip/o is the word root-combining form for _____.

lip/oma
lipoma
li po' ma

17
A fatty tumor is called a

_____ / _____ .

18
Carcin/o is the word root-combining form for

cancer. A carcin/oma is a ** _____

cancerous or
  malignant tumor

_____ .

carcin/oma
carcinoma
car si no' ma

19
A carcinoma may occur in almost any part of
the body. A stomach cancer is called gastric

_____ / _____ .

20
Cancer of the spleen is called splenic

carcinoma

_____ . Cancer of the tonsil is

carcinoma

tonsillar _____ . Cancer of

duodenal
  carcinoma

the duodenum is called * _____

_____ .

lip/oid
lipoid
lip' oid

21
Lipoma is a fatty tumor; oid is a suffix which
means like or resembling. Build a word that
means fatlike or resembling fat:

_____ / _____ .

22

The word lipoid is used in chemistry or pathology. It describes a substance that looks like fat, dissolves like fat, but is not fat. Cholesterol is an alcohol that resembles fat; therefore

lipoid   it is a _____.

23

muc/oid   Muc/oid means resembling mucus. There is a
mucoid   substance in connective tissue that resembles
mu' koyd
                          mucus. This is a _____/_____ substance.

24

                          There is a protein in the body that is said to be
                          mucoid in nature.   Mucoid means
resembling
  mucus   *_____.

25

                          Anything that resembles mucus is called a

mucoid   _____.

26

                          The larynx contains the vocal cords. Laryng/o
                          is used to build words that refer to the larynx.
laryng/itis   Form a word that means inflammation of the
laryngitis
lar in ji' tis   larynx: _____/_____.

27

                          After a bad cold a patient may develop laryngi-

                          tis, which means **_____
inflammation of
  the larynx   _____.

28

                          Laryng/ostomy means making a new opening
                          into the larynx. When another source of air is
laryng/ostomy   needed for breathing or speaking, a
laryngostomy
lar in gos' to mi   _____/_____ is done.

29
The meaning of ostomy is the creation of a new opening that will be permanent. When a permanent opening has been made through the neck

laryngostomy

into the larynx, a _____ has been performed.

30

ostomy

The word ending for new opening is _____.

31

laryng/otomy
laryngotomy
lar in got' o mi

When a temporary opening is wanted into the larynx, the surgical procedure is a laryng/otomy. An incision into the larynx is called a

_____/_____.

32
When a patient has pneumonia and a freer flow of air is needed temporarily, the surgeon may incise the larynx and thus do a

laryngotomy

_____.

33
The word ending that means making a temporary incision is _____.

otomy

34
At this stage of word building, students sometimes find that they have one big headache. The word for pain in the head is cephal/algia. The

cephal

word root for head is _____.

35
If you are now suffering from a headache, persevere, for later this gets to be fun. Any pain in the head may be called

cephal/algia
cephalalgia
sef a lal' ji a

_____/_____.

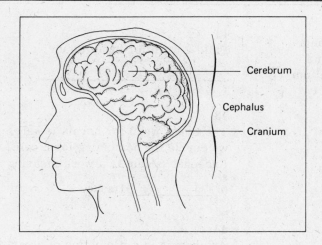

36
The word root-combining form for head is
cephal/o. The word for pain in the head is

cephalalgia

_____.

37
headache   Cephalalgia means _____.

38
Cephal/ic means pertaining to or toward the

adjective   head. Cephal/ic is a (an) _____
                        (noun/adjective). This is evident because

ic   cephalic ends in _____.

39
A case history reporting head cuts due to an

cephal/ic
cephalic   accident might read, "_____/_____
sef al' ic   lacerations present."

40
A tumor located on the head might be noted as

cephalic   a _____ tumor.

41
Inside the head, enclosed in bone, is the brain.
Encephal/o is used in words pertaining to the

encephal/itis   brain. Build a word meaning inflammation of
encephalitis
en sef a li' tis   the brain: _____/_____.

encephal/oma
encephaloma
en sef al o' ma

42
Build a word for brain tumor:

_____ / _____ .

43
The Greek word for hernia is <u>kele</u>. From this
we derive the combining form cele/o or o/cele.
Encephal/o/cele is a word meaning herniation

brain

of _____ tissue.

encephal/o/cele
encephalocele
en sef' al o sēl

44
Any hernia is a projection of a part from its
natural cavity. Herniation is indicated by cele.
A projection of brain tissue from its natural

cavity is an _____ / __ / _____ .

encephalocele

45
Fluid inside the head sometimes causes
herniation. The symptom in medical language

is called an _____ .

46
Malac/ia is a word meaning softening of a
tissue. Encephal/o/malac/ia means

softening of
brain tissue

** _____

_____ .

encephal/o/
malac/ia
encephalomalacia
en sef al o mal
a' si a

47
Malac/o is the combining form. A noun meaning softening of brain tissue is

_____ / __ / _____ / ____ .

encephalomalacia

48
An accident that causes brain injury could result in the softening of some brain tissue or

_____ .

49
oste/itis
osteitis
os te i' tis

Oste/o is the combining form referring to bone.
A word meaning inflammation of the bone is

_____/_____ .

50
softening
  of bones

What do you think oste/o/malac/ia means ?

** _____ .

51
oste/o/malac/ia
osteomalacia
os te o mal a' si a

When calcium leaves the bones and they lose
some of their hardness, the disorder is called

_____/ /_____ /____ .

52
osteomalacia

A disorder of the parathyroid gland can cause
calcium to be withdrawn from the bones. When

this occurs, _____ results.

53
oste/oma
osteoma
os te o' ma

A hard outgrowth on a bone may be a bone tumor. In medical terminology, it would be re-

ferred to as an _____/_____ .

54
surgical repair
  of a joint

Arthr/o refers to joints; plast/y means surgical repair of. What does arthr/o/plast/y

mean? ** _____

_____ .

55
arthr/o/plast/y
arthroplasty
ar' thro plas ti

Think of a plast/ic surgeon building a new nose
or doing a face lifting. These are surgical re-
pairs. When a joint has lost its ability to move,
movement can sometimes be restored by an

_____/ /_____ /____ .

56

If a child is born without a joint, sometimes one can be formed for him by a surgical procedure

arthroplasty   called _____.

arthr/itis   **57**
arthritis   Form a word that means inflammation of a
ar thri' tis   joint: _____/_____.

arthr/otomy   **58**
arthrotomy   Now form a word that means incision into a
arth rot' o mi   joint: _____/_____

59

The word oste/o/chondr/itis means inflammation of the bone and cartilage. The word root-combining form for cartilage must be

chondr/o   _____/o.

60

Analyze oste/o/chondr/itis:

oste/o   _____/___   combining form for bone,

chondr   _____ word root for cartilage,

itis   _____   suffix for inflammation.

oste/o/chondr/itis   Now put all the parts together:
osteochondritis
os te o kon dri' tis   _____/ /_____/_____.

inflammation of bone   What does it mean? **_____
  and cartilage
                                _____

excision of   **61**
  cartilage   Chondr/ectomy means ** _____

                                _____.

62
Cost/al forms words that mean pertaining to the ribs. Inter/cost/al means between the ribs.

inter

The prefix for between is _____.

63
inter/cost/al
intercostal
in ter kos' tal

There are short, strong muscles between the ribs. These muscles move the ribs in breath-

ing and are called _____/_____/_____ muscles.

64
One set of between-the-ribs muscles enlarges the rib cage when breathing in. When exhaling, the rib cage is made smaller by another set of

intercostal

_____ muscles.
(between-the-ribs)

65
teeth

A dent/ist takes care of _____. A dent/

teeth

ifrice is used for cleaning _____.

66
between the
  teeth

Inter/dent/al means ** _____

_____. An inter/dental activity

between the
  teeth

occurs ** _____

_____.

67
Inter/dent/al is an adjective and must modify a noun. "Interdental spaces" means

spaces between
  the teeth

** _____

_____.

68
Try making a few new words. A cavity between

interdental

the teeth is called an _____ cavity.

dent/algia
dentalgia
den tal' ji a

69

Pain in the teeth, or a toothache, is called

_____/_____.

dent/oid
dentoid
den' toid

70

Form a word that means tooth-shaped or re-

sembling a tooth: _____/_____.

Below are 30 of the medical terms you formed in Unit 2. Read them one at a time and pronounce each aloud.

adenectomy	chondritis	intercostal
adenitis	dental	laryngitis
adenoma	dentalgia	laryngostomy
arthritis	dentoid	lipoid
arthroplasty	encephalitis	lipoma
arthrotomy	encephalocele	mucoid
carcinoma	encephaloma	osteitis
cephalalgia	hyperemesis	osteoma
cephalic	hypertrophy	osteomalacia
chondrectomy	hypodermic	thyroidectomy

Before going on to the next unit take the Unit 2 Self-Test.

UNIT 2   SELF-TEST

PART 1

From the list on the right select the correct meaning for each of the
following terms. Write the letters in the space provided.

_____	1. Osteomalacia	a. Overdevelopment
_____	2. Adenoma	b. A needle inserted under the skin
_____	3. Intercostal	c. Surgical removal of cartilage
_____	4. Laryngotomy	d. Between the ribs
_____	5. Cephalalgia	e. Surgical repair of a joint
_____	6. Chondrectomy	f. Softening of bone tissue
_____	7. Encephalocele	g. Herniation of the brain tissue inside of the head
_____	8. Hypertrophy	
_____	9. Arthroplasty	h. Tumor of glandular tissue
_____	10. Hypodermic	i. Headache
		j. Incision into the larynx

PART 2

Complete each of the medical terms on the right with the appropriate
prefix and/or suffix:

1. Surgical removal of the thyroid gland   Thyroid _____

2. Inflammation of glandular tissue   Aden _____

3. A malignant tumor   Carcin _____

4. Excessive vomiting   _____ emesis

5. Resembling mucus   Muc _____

6. Toothache   _____ algia

7. Making a new permanent opening
   into the larynx   Laryng _____

8. Inflammation of inside the head   _____ cephal _____

9. A tumor of fat tissue   _____ oma

10. Pertaining to the teeth   Dent _____

ANSWERS

Part 1	Part 2
1. f	1. Thyroidectomy
2. h	2. Adenitis
3. d	3. Carcinoma
4. j	4. Hyperemesis
5. i	5. Mucoid
6. c	6. Dentalgia
7. g	7. Laryngostomy
8. a	8. Encephalitis
9. e	9. Lipoma
10. b	10. Dental

Unit 3

In Unit 3 you will put together at least 50 new words, using the following word root-combining forms, prefixes, and suffixes.

abdomin/o (abdomen)
centesis (puncture)
cerebr/o (cerebrum)
chol/e (bile, gall)
cocc/i (coccus)
crani/o (cranium)
cyst/o (bladder, sac)
hydr/o (water)
lith/o (stone, calculus)
lumb/o (loin)

metr/o, meter (measure)
ot/o (ear)
pelv/i (pelvis)
phob/ia (fear)
pub/o (pubis)
py/o (pus)
rhin/o (nose)
therap/o (treatment)
thorac/o (thorax)

ab- (away from)
ad- (toward)
supra- (above)

-ar (pertaining to)
-scope, -scopy (examining)
-orrhea (flow)
-meter (measuring instrument)
-genesis, gen/o (development, formation)

	1
	The prefix ab means from or away from.
away from	Abnormal means * _____ normal.

	2
from or away from	The prefix ab means ** _____ _____ .

35

3
Ab/errant uses the prefix ab before the English word for wandering.   Ab/errant means

wandering from
(the normal
course of events)

** _____.

4
Ab/errant is used in medicine to describe a structure that wanders from the normal. When some nerve fibers follow an unusual route, they

ab/errant
aberrant
ab er' ant

form an _____/_____ nerve.

5
Aberrant nerves wander from the normal nerve track. Blood vessels that follow a path of their

aberrant

own are _____ vessels.

6
Ab/duct/ion means movement away from a mid-line. When the hand is raised from the side of

ab/duct/ion
abduction
ab duc' shun

the body, ____/_____/_____ has occurred.

7
Abduction can occur from any midline. When the fingers of the hand are spread apart,

abduction

_____ has occurred in four fingers.

8
When a child has been kidnapped and taken from

abducted

his parents, he has been _____ (past tense verb).

9
On the other hand, ad is a prefix meaning toward. Movement toward a midline is

ad/duction
adduction
ad duc' shun

_____/_____.

10

ab

The prefix meaning from or away from is ____.
The prefix meaning toward, or toward the mid-

ad

line, is ____.

11

When two normally separate tissues join together, they adhere to each other like adhesive
tape.   Underline the part of the word that means

ad/<u>hesion</u>

sticking or joining: ad/hesion.

12

ad/hesion
adhesion
ad he' shun

Several years ago patients did not walk
soon enough after surgery, which sometimes
resulted in abnormal joining of tissues to
each other. Write the word that means the joining
and healing together of tissues.   ____/_____

13

Now patients walk the day following an appen-
dectomy.   This has nearly eliminated

adhesions

_____.

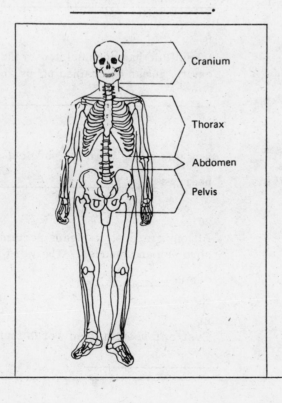

Cranium

Thorax

Abdomen

Pelvis

14
Abdomin/o is used to form words about the
abdomen. When you see abdomin/o in a word,

abdomen
ab do' men

you think of the _____.

15
Abdomin/al is an adjective that means

pertaining to
  the abdomen

** _____.

16
Abdomin/o/centesis means tapping or punctur-
ing the abdomen. This is a surgical puncture.
The word for surgical puncture of the abdomen

abdomin/o/
  centesis
abdominocentesis
ab dom i no sen
  ti' sis

is _____ / / _____.

17
Centesis (surgical puncture) is a word in itself.
Build a word meaning surgical puncture or
puncturing or tapping of the abdomen:

abdominocentesis

_____.

18
When fluid has accumulated in the abdomin/al
cavity, it can be drained off by an

abdominocentesis

_____.

19
Try this. The word for surgical puncture of the

cardi/o/centesis
cardiocentesis
kar di o sen ti' sis

heart is _____ / / _____.

20
Abdomin/o/cyst/ic means pertaining to the
abdomen and bladder. The word root for blad-

cyst

der is _____.

21
Cyst/o is used to form words that refer to the

bladder

_____.

22

To refer to the urinary bladder or any sac containing fluid use some form of _____ / ___.

cyst/o

23

cyst/otomy
cystotomy
sis tot' o mi

The word for incision into the bladder is

_____ / _____.

cyst/itis
cystitis
sis ti' tis

Inflammation of the bladder is

_____ / _____.

cyst/ectomy
cystectomy
sis tek' to mi

The word for excision of the bladder is

_____ / _____.

24

The chest is referred to as the thorax. What does abdomin/o/thorac/ic mean?

pertaining to
  the abdomen
  and thorax

** _____

_____.

abdomin/o/thorac/ic
abdominothoracic
ab dom i no tho
  ras' ic

25

A word that means, literally, pertaining to the abdomen and chest is

_____ / / _____ / ___.

26

thorac/ic
thoracic
thor as' ik

Thorac/o is used to form words about the thorax or chest. A word that means pertaining

to the chest is _____ / ___.

thorac/otomy
thoracotomy
tho rak ot' o mi

Write a word that means incision of the chest:

_____ / _____.

thorac/o/centesis
thoracocentesis
tho rak o sen ti' sis

Write a word that means surgical tapping of the chest to remove fluids:

_____ / / _____.

thorac/o/plast/y
thoracoplasty
tho' ra ko plas ti

A word for surgical repair of the chest is

_____ / / plast / y .

cyst/o/plast/y
cystoplasty
sis' to plas ti

Now write a word for surgical repair of the bladder:

_____ / / _____ / __.

27
A hydr/o/cyst is a sac (or bladder) filled with watery fluid. Hydr/o is used in words to

water, fluid, or
    watery fluid

mean _____.

28
What does hydr/o/cephal/us mean?

** _____

a collection of
    fluid in the head

_____.

29
A disease characterized by an enlarged head due to increased amount of fluid in the skull is

hydr/o/cephal/us
hydrocephalus
hi dro sef' a lus

called _____ / / _____ / __.

30
Unless arrested, this disease results in deformity. The face seems small. The eyes are abnormal. The head is large and brain damage

hydrocephalus

may be a result of _____.

31
Hydr/o/phob/ia means having an abnormal fear of water. Phob/ia means

abnormal fear

* _____.

32
An abnormal fear of water is

hydr/o/phob/ia
hydrophobia
hi dro fo' bi a

_____ / / _____ / __.

33

Some parents are abnormally afraid to have
their children swim or even ride in a boat.

hydrophobia   These parents suffer from _____.

hydr/o/therap/y   34
hydrotherapy   Therap/y means treatment.   Treatment by
hi dro ther' a pi   water is _____ / ____ / _____ / __.

35
Swirling water baths are a form of

hydrotherapy   _____.

36
Lumb/o builds words about the loin or lower
back. An adjective which means pertaining to

lumb   the loin is _____ / ar .

37
There are five vertebrae in the lower back
lumb/ar
lumbar   (loin area) which are called _____ / ____
lum' bar   vertebrae.

pertaining to the   38
chest and loin   Thorac/o/lumb/ar means ** _____
(or equivalent)
_____.

39
Supra/lumb/ar means above the lumbar region.
What is the prefix that means above?

supra   _____.

above the lumbar   40
region or above   Supra/lumb/ar means ** _____
the loin
_____.

Supra/cost/al means ** _____

above the ribs   _____.

41
The pub/is is a bone of the pelvis. Pub/is is

noun

a (an) _____ (noun/adjective).

pubic

What is the adjectival form? _____.

42
The suprapubic region is above the arch of the
pub/is. When the abdomen is incised above the

supra/pub/ic
suprapubic
su pra pu' bik

pubis, an incision is made in the

_____ / _____ / _____ region.

43
anything close to:
   incision of bladder
   from the supra-
   pubic region

Try to figure out what surgery is done in a

supra/pubic cyst/otomy. ** _____ _____

_____.

44
The pelvis is formed by the pelvic bones. During pregnancy, to find the measurement of a
woman's pelvis, the physician does pelv/i/
metr/y. What part of the word refers to mea-

metr

surement of? _____.

45
To determine whether a woman has a pelvis
large enough to avoid trouble during labor, a

pelvimetry
pel vim' et ri

physician can do _____.

46
What do you think pelvimeter means?

a measuring device
   used for pelvimetry
   (or equivalent)

**
_____

_____.

47
When the physician measures the patient's pel-

pelvimetry

vis, he does _____.

pelvimeter

The instrument he uses is a _____.

supra/pelv/ic suprapelvic su pra pel' vic	**48** Give the adjective meaning above the pelvis: _____/_____/____ .
surgical repair of the skull or cranium	**49** Crani/o is used in words referring to the crani/um or skull. Crani/o/plast/y means ** _____ _____.
crani/ectomy craniectomy kra ni ek' to mi	**50** Write a medical term for each of the following: excision of part of the cranium, _____/_____;
crani/otomy craniotomy kra ni ot' o mi	incision into the skull _____/_____;
crani/o/meter craniometer kra ni om' et er	an instrument to measure the cranium, _____/_/_____.
of or pertaining to the cerebrum and skull (cranium)	**51** The cerebrum (cerebr/o) is the part of the brain in which thought occurs. What is the meaning of crani/o/cerebr/al? ** _____ _____.
cerebrum ser' e brum	**52** Thinking, feeling, and movement are controlled by the gray matter of the _____. (Have you ever been told to use your "gray matter"? This is why.)
cerebr/al cerebral ser' e bral	**53** The adjectival form of cerebrum is _____/____.

54

spin/al
spinal
spi' nal

Cerebr/o/spin/al refers to the brain and spinal cord. What part of the word means pertaining to the spinal cord? _____/_____.

55

cerebr/o/spin/al
cerebrospinal
ser e bro spi' nal

A puncture or tap to remove fluid from the area around the cerebrum and spinal cord is called a _____/ /_____/_____ puncture.

56

Let's try some different ones. Cocc/i is the plural of cocc/us. When building words about a whole family of bacteria, the cocci, use the

cocc

word root _____.

57

Pneumonia is caused by the pneumococcus. From this you know that the germ responsible

cocc/i
kok' si

for pneumonia belongs to the family _____/ (plural).

58

There are three main types of coccus:

cocci growing in pairs are

dipl/o/cocc/i

_dipl____/ o /_____/___;

cocci growing in twisted chains are

strept/o/cocc/i

strept/ o /_____/___;

cocci growing in clusters are

staphyl/o/cocc/i

staphyl/ o /_____/___.

59

If you should see a twisted chain of cocci when examining a slide under a microscope, you would

strept/o/cocc/i

say they were _____/ /_____/___.

60

Staphyle is the Greek word for bunch of grapes.
If you should see a cluster of cocci when using
a microscope, you would say they
were

staphyl/o/cocc/i
staphylococci
staf il o kok' si

_____ / / _____ / __ .

61

The bacteria that cause carbuncles grow in
clusters like a bunch of grapes. Carbuncles

staphylococci

are caused by _____ .

62

Py/o is the word root-combining form used for
words involving pus. Genesis (gen/o) is from a
Greek word meaning formation or development.

Py/o/gen/ic means ** _____

producing pus

_____ .

py/o/gen/ic
pyogenic
pi o jen' ik

63

Staphylococci produce pus; therefore they are

referred to as _____ / / _____ / __ .

64

Bacteria that form pus are referred to as

pyogenic

_____ (adjective).

65

Boils become purulent (contain pus). This pus

pyogenic

if formed by _____ bacteria.

66

A combining form that you will use as a suffix
is orrhea; orrhea ends a word and it follows a
word root. It means flow or discharge.

Py/orrhea means ** _____

discharge of pus

_____ .

py/orrhea
pyorrhea
pi o re' a

67
The suffix orrhea refers to any flow or discharge. A discharge or flow of pus is called

_____/_____.

pyorrhea

68
Pyorrhea alveolaris is a disease of the teeth and gums. The part of this disease's name that tells you that pus is discharged is

_____.

pyorrhea

69
There is also a disease of the salivary gland symptomized by the flow of pus. This is

_____ salivaris.

ear

70
Ot/orrhea means a discharging ear; ot/o is the word root-combining form for _____.

ot/orrhea
otorrhea
o to re' a

71
Ot/orrhea is both a symptom and a disease. No matter which is meant, the word

_____/_____ is used.

otorrhea

72
This disease involves discharge, inflammation, and deafness. One of its symptoms is also its name, _____.

inflammation of
   the middle ear

73
Ot/itis media may be the cause of otorrhea.

Ot/itis media means ** _____

_____.

ot/algia
otalgia
o tal' ji a

74
Otitis usually causes ear pain, which in medical terminology we call _____ / _____ .

otalgia

75
Small children often complain of earache.
Medically this could be called _____ .

nose

76
Rhinorrhea means discharge from the nose.
Rhin/o is used in words about the _____ .

rhin/itis
rhinitis
ri ni' tis

rhin/orrhea
rhinorrhea
ri no re' a

77
Taking what is necessary from rhin/o, form a
word that means inflammation of the nose:

_____ / _____ .

Drainage from the nose due to a head cold is a

symptom called _____ / _____ .

rhinorrhea

78
A discharge from the sinuses through the nose
is a form of _____ .

rhin/o/plast/y
rhinoplasty
ri' no plas ti

rhin/otomy
rhinotomy
ri not' o mi

79
Build a word that means surgical repair of the

nose: _____ / / _____ / __ .

Form one that means incision of the nose:

_____ / _____ .

calculus
  or stone

80
A rhin/o/lith is a calculus or stone in the nose.
Lith/o is the combining form for

** _____ .

calculi (calculus) or stones	**81** Lithogenesis means producing or forming **_____** .
lith/otomy lithotomy lith ot' o mi	**82** Taking what is necessary from lith/o, build a word meaning an incision for the removal of a stone: _____ / _____ .
gall or bile	**83** Calculi or stones can be formed in many places in the body. A chol/e/lith is a gallstone. Chol/e is the word root-combining form for _____ .
chol/e/lith cholelith ko' le lith	**84** One cause of gallbladder disease is the pres- ence of a gallstone or _____ / / _____ .
cholelith	**85** No matter what the size or shape, irritation and blockage of the gallbladder can be caused by a _____ .
gallbladder	**86** Gall is the fluid secreted by the gallbladder. Chol/e/cyst is a medical name for the _____ .
chol/e/cyst/itis cholecystitis ko le sis ti' tis	**87** When gallstones result in inflammation of the gallbladder (chol/e/cyst), medically this con- dition is called _____ / / _____ / _____ .

88

Cholecystitis is accompanied by pain and hyperemesis. Fatty foods aggravate these symptoms
and should be avoided in cases of

cholecystitis

_____.

89

Butter, cream, and even whole milk contain
fat and should be avoided by patients with

cholecystitis

_____.

chol/e/cyst/otomy
cholecystotomy
ko le sis tot' o mi
  or
chol/e/lith/otomy
cholelithotomy
kol e lith ot' o mi

90

When a cholelith causes cholecystitis, one of
two surgical procedures may be needed. One
is an incision into the gallbladder, a

_____ / / _____ / _____.

91

Usually the presence of a gallstone calls for
the excision of the gallbladder. This is a

chol/e/cyst/ectomy
cholecystectomy
ko le sis tekt' o mi

_____ / _____ / _____.

rhin/o/lith
rhinolith
ri' no lith

A calculus or stone in the nose is a

_____ / / _____.

92

In the following rules and examples you will
find additional material to help you with word
building. The chances are fifty-fifty that by
now you have figured out a system concerning
the order in which word parts go together. If
you have, you may skip this material. If you
have not, study the examples; they will help
you.

RULE I: About 90 percent of the time the part of the word that is indicated first comes last.

Examples

1. Inflammation of the bladder

inflammation	/	itis
(of the) bladder	cyst /	
cyst	/ itis	

2. One who specializes in skin disorders

one who specializes (studies)	/	/logist
(in) skin (disorders)	dermat / o /	
dermat	/ o /logist	

3. Pertaining to the abdomen and bladder

pertaining to	/	/	/ic
(the) abdomen	abdomin / o /		/
(and) bladder	/	/ cyst /	
abdomin	/ o / cyst /ic		

RULE II: When body systems are involved, words are usually built in order of organs passed in going through the system. (The first part still comes last.)

Examples

1. Inflammation of the stomach and small intestine

inflammation	/	/	/itis
(of the) stomach	gastr / o /		/
(and) small intestine	/	/ enter /	
gastr	/ o / enter /itis		

2. Removal of the uterus, fallopian tubes, and ovaries

removal of	/ /	/ /	/ectomy	
(the) uterus	hyster /o/	/ /	/	
fallopian tubes	/ /salping /o/		/	
(and) ovaries	/ /	/ /-oophor /		
hyster /o/ salping /o/-oophor /ectomy				

Of course, prefixes still come in front of the word.

Below are 40 of the new medical terms you formed in Unit 3. Read them one at a time and pronounce each aloud.

aberrant	craniotomy	pelvic
abdominal	cranium	pelvimetry
abdominocentesis	cystitis	pyogenic
abduction	cystocele	pyorrhea
adduction	cystotomy	rhinitis
cardiocentesis	diplococci	rhinoplasty
cerebral	hydrocephalus	rhinorrhea
cerebrospinal	hydrotherapy	staphylococci
cerebrum	lithotomy	suprapubic
cholecystectomy	lumbar	thoracocentesis
cholecystitis	otalgia	thoracic
cholelithotomy	otitis	thoracoplasty
craniectomy	otorrhea	thoracotomy
cranioplasty		

Take the Unit 3 Self-Test before going on.

UNIT 3   SELF-TEST

From the list on the right select the correct meaning for each of the
following terms. Write the letter in the space provided.

_____	1.	Thoracocentesis	a. Pertaining to the cerebrum and spinal cord
_____	2.	Cholelithotomy	
_____	3.	Otorrhea	b. Relating to the pubis
_____	4.	Cystotomy	c. Wandering or out of the normal place
_____	5.	Suprapelvic	
_____	6.	Cranium	d. Tapping or puncturing the chest cavity
_____	7.	Cerebrospinal	e. Movement toward the midline
_____	8.	Hydrophobia	f. Abnormal fear of water
_____	9.	Adduction	g. Running or draining from the ear
_____	10.	Streptococci	h. Incision into the bladder
_____	11.	Pyogenic	i. Producing pus
_____	12.	Aberrant	j. The bony vault surrounding the brain
_____	13.	Pubic	
_____	14.	Cholecystotomy	k. Incision for the purpose of removing a gallstone
_____	15.	Cystoplasty	l. Relating to above the pelvis
			m. Cocci bacteria that grow in chains
			n. Surgical repair of the bladder
			o. Incision into the gall bladder

PART 2

Complete each of the medical terms on the right with the appropriate word root-combining form:

1. Herniation of the bladder _____ cele

2. Tapping or puncturing the heart _____ centesis

3. Surgical repair of the bony vault that encloses the brain _____ plasty

4. Earache _____ algia

5. Gallstone _____ lith

6. Inflammation of the nose _____ itis

7. Measurement of the pelvis _____ metry

8. Relating to the thorax and the loin area _____ lumbar

9. Collection of fluid in the head Hydro _____ us

10. Incision into the cranium _____ otomy

11. Relating to above the pubis Supra _____ ic

12. Surgical repair of the chest _____ plasty

13. Instrument for measuring the pelvis _____ meter

14. Relating to the abdomen _____ al

15. Surgical removal of the gallbladder Chole _____ ectomy

ANSWERS

Part 1

1.	d	9.	e
2.	k	10.	m
3.	g	11.	i
4.	h	12.	c
5.	l	13.	b
6.	j	14.	o
7.	a	15.	n
8.	f		

Part 2

1. Cystocele
2. Cardiocentesis
3. Cranioplasty
4. Otalgia
5. Cholelith
6. Rhinitis
7. Pelvimetry
8. Thoracolumbar
9. Hydrocephalus
10. Craniotomy
11. Suprapubic
12. Thoracoplasty
13. Pelvimeter
14. Abdominal
15. Cholecystectomy

Unit 4

In Unit 4 you will make at least 60 new words by using some of the word root-combining forms, prefixes, and suffixes you have covered in earlier units. You will also use the following:

angi/o (vessel)
arter/i/o (artery)
blast/o (embryo)
blephar/o (eyelid)
fibr/o (fiber)
hem/o, hemat/o (blood)
hyster/o (uterus)
kinesi/o (motion)
lys/o (destruction)
melan/o (black)
my/o (muscle)
nephr/o (kidney)

neur/o (nerve)
oophor/o (ovary)
peps/o, peps/ia (digestion)
pne/o (air, breathe)
pneum/o, pneumon/o (lung)
pyel/o (pelvis of the kidney)
salping/o (fallopian tube)
scler/o (tough, hard)
spermat/o (sperm)
ureter/o (ureter)
urethr/o (urethra)
ur/o (urine)

a-, an- (without)
brady- (slow)
dys- (pain)
tachy- (fast)

-blast (embryonic)
-ia (noun ending)
-orrhaphy (suture)
-orrhagia (hemorrhage)
-pexy (fixation)
-ptosis (drooping)
-spasm (twitching)
-sperm (sperm)

1
Brad/y is used in words to mean slow. Brad/y/

slow   cardi/a means _____ heart action.

brad/y/cardi/a
bradycardia
brad i kar' di a

2
Abnormally slow heart action is

_____ / / _____ / ___ .

3
Kinesi/o is used in words to mean movement
or motion. Brad/y/kinesi/a means

** _____

slowness of
  movement

_____ .

pain on movement
  or movement pain

4
Kinesi/algia means ** _____

_____ .

kinesi/algia
kinesialgia
ki ne si al' ji a

5
When you have to move any sore or injured
part of the body, pain occurs. Moving a bro-
ken arm causes _____ / _____ .

kinesialgia

6
After a first ride on horseback almost any

movement causes _____ .

kinesi/o/logy
kinesiology
kin es i ol' o ji

7
The suffix ology means study of. (Remember
o/logist?) The study of muscular movements

is _____ / / _____ .

kinesiology

8
Kinesi/o/logy is the study of movement. The
study of muscular movement during exercise
would be done in the field of

_____ .

kinesiology

9
The whole science of how the body moves is

embraced in the field of _____ .

10
Brad/y/kinesi/a means ** _____

abnormally slow
  movement

_____.

11
Tach/y is used in words to show the opposite
of slow. Thus tach/y /card/ia means

abnormally fast
  or rapid heart
  action

** _____

_____.

tach/y/cardi/a
tachycardia
tak i kar' di a

12
Write the medical term for an abnormally fast

heartbeat: _____ / / _____ / ___.

13
Pne/o comes from the Greek word <u>pneia</u>
(breathe). Pne/o any place in a word means

breathe or
  breathing

_____.

14
When pne/o begins a word, the "p" is silent.
When pne/o occurs later in a word, it is pro-
nounced; for example, when you pronounce

will
(brad ip ne' a)

brad/y/pne/a, you _____ pronounce
                  (will/ will not)
the "p." In the term pne/u/mon/ia, the "p" is

silent

_____.
(pronounced/silent)

15
Brad/y/pne/a means ** _____

slow breathing

_____.

tach/y/pne/a
tachypnea
tak ip ne' a

A word for rapid breathing is

_____ / / _____ / ___.

16

The rate of respiration (breathing) is controlled by the amount of carbon dioxide in the blood. Increased carbon dioxide speeds up breathing

tachypnea   and causes _____.

17

Muscle exercise increases the amount of carbon dioxide in the blood. This speeds respiration

tachypnea   tion and produces _____.

18

The prefix <u>a</u> literally means without. Thus

apnea means ** _____

without breathing   _____.

19

A/pnea really means temporary cessation of breathing. If the failure to breathe were not temporary, death would result. Temporary

a/pne/a   cessation of breathing is referred to as
apnea
ap ne' a   ____/_____/___.

20

If the level of carbon dioxide in the blood falls very low, temporary cessation of breathing

apnea   results. This is called _____.

21

If breathing is merely very slow, it is called

bradypnea   _____.

22

When breathing is abnormally fast, it is called

tachypnea   _____. The prefix meaning

a   without is _____.

23

dys/pne/a
dyspnea
disp ne' a

The prefix dys means painful, bad, or difficult.
Dys/troph/y literally means bad development.
Write a word for difficult breathing:

_____/_____/__.

24

Dys/men/orrhea means painful menstruation.
The prefix for painful, bad, or difficult is

dys

_____.

25

Pepsis (peps/o) is the Greek word for diges-

poor or painful
  digestion

tion. Dys/peps/ia means ** _____

_____.

26

dys/peps/ia
dyspepsia
dis pep' si a

Eating under tension may cause painful or poor

digestion. This is called _____/_____/__.

27

Contemplating the troubles of the world when

dyspepsia

eating is a good cause for _____.

28

Refer to the chart on the following page when
working frames 29 through 38.

COMBINING FORM	COMBINING FORM	SUFFIX
my/o (muscle)	spasm o/spasm/o (twitch, twitching)	spasm (word in itself)

	blast
	o/blast/o
	(germ or embryonic;
	  gives rise to some-
	  thing else)
		blast
		(word in itself)

angi/o (vessel)	scler/o (hard)	osis (use with scler/o)
	fibr/o (fibrous, fiber)	oma (use with fibr/o)
neur/o (nerve or neuron)	lys/o (breaking down, destruction)	is-noun suffix (use with lys/o)

29

neur/o/blast
neuroblast
nu' ro blast

An embryonic (germ) cell from which a muscle develops is a my/o/blast. A germ cell from which a nerve cell develops is a

_____/ /_____.

angi/o/blast
angioblast
an' ji o blast

A germ cell from which vessels develop is an

_____/ /_____.

30

my/o/spasm
myospasm
mi' o spazm

A spasm of a nerve is a neur/o/spasm. A spasm of a muscle is a

_____/ /_____.

angi/o/spasm
angiospasm
an' ji o spazm

A spasm of a vessel is an

_____/ /_____.

31

angi/o/scler/osis
angiosclerosis
an ji o skler o' sis

A (condition of) hardening of nerve tissue is neur/o/scler/osis. A hardening of a vessel

is _____/____/_____/_____.

my/o/scler/osis
myosclerosis
mi o skler o' sis

A hardening of muscle tissue is

_____/____/_____/_____.

32

neur/o/fibr/oma
neurofibroma
nu ro fi bro' ma

A tumor containing muscle fibers is a my/o/fibr/oma. A tumor containing nerve

fibers is a _____/____/_____/_____.

angi/o/fibr/oma
angiofibroma
an ji o fi bro' ma

A vessel tumor containing fibers is an

_____/____/_____/_____.

33

neur/o/lys/is
neurolysis
nu rol' i sis

The destruction of muscle tissue is my/o/lys/is. The destruction of nerve tissue is

_____/____/_____/_____.

angi/o/lys/is
angiolysis
an ji ol' i sis

The destruction or breaking down of vessels is

_____/____/_____/_____.

34

arteri/o/scler/osis
arteriosclerosis
ar te ri o skler
  o' sis

Refer to the chart only when you must.
Arteri/o is used in words about the arteries.
A word meaning hardening of the arteries is

_____/____/_____/_____

arteri/o/fibr/osis
arteriofibrosis
ar te ri o fi bro' sis

Build a word meaning a fibrous condition of the arteries:

_____/____/_____/_____.

arteri/o/malac/ia
arteriomalacia
ar te ri o ma la' ci a

A softening of the arteries is called:

_____/_____/_____.

arteri/o/spasm
arteriospasm
ar te' ri o spazm

Build a word meaning arterial spasm:

_____/____/_____.

lip/o/lys/is
lipolysis
lip ol' i sis

Destruction (breakdown) of fat is called

_____/___/_____/_____.

35
Hem/o refers to blood. A tumor of a blood
vessel is a hem/angi/oma. (Note dropped o.)

hem/angi/itis
hemangiitis
hem an ji i' tis

An inflammation of a blood vessel is

_____/_____/_____.

hem/o/lys/is
hemolysis
hem ol' is is

Destruction of blood tissue (cells) is

_____/___/_____/____.

36
Hemat/o also refers to blood. The study of

hemat/o/log/y
hematology
hem at ol' o gi

blood is _____/___/_____/___.

hemat/o/log/ist
hematologist
hem at ol' o gist

One who specializes in the science of blood is

a _____/___/_____/_____.

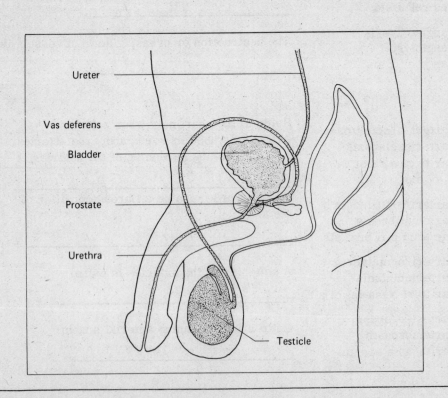

Ureter

Vas deferens

Bladder

Prostate

Urethra

Testicle

37
<u>Sperma</u> is the Greek word meaning seed.
Spermat/o is used in words about spermat/o/
zoa or male germ cells (sperm). Spermat/o/

formation of sperma-
tozoa, sperm, or
male germ cells

genesis means ** _____

_____ .

38
Give a word meaning:
the destruction of spermatozoa,

spermat/o/lys/is
spermatolysis
sper mat ol' i sis

_____ / / _____ / ____ ;

spermat/o/blast
spermatoblast
sper mat' o blast

an embryonic male cell,

_____ / / _____ ;

spermat/oid
spermatoid
sper' mat oyd

resembling sperm,

_____ / _____ .

39
Summarize what you learned in frames 29 to
38:

muscle   my/o   means _____ ,
vessel   angi/o   means _____ ,
nerve   neur/o   means _____ ,

40
twitching   spasm   means _____ ,
germ or embryonic blast/o   means _____ ,
hard   scler/o   means _____ ,
fibrous   fibr/o   means _____ ,
destruction   lys/o   means _____ ,

41

spermatozoa (sperm)	spermat/o	means	_____ ,
blood	hemat/o	means	_____ ,
blood	hem/o	means	_____ ,
formation	genesis	means	_____ .

Correct any definitions you may have missed; then cover the word roots, read the definitions you have written, and write the appropriate word root in the right-hand margin.

42
The Greek word for egg is <u>oon</u>. In scientific words o/o (pronounce both o's) means egg or

an embryonic egg
   cell (a cell that will
become an ovum)

ovum. An o/o/blast is ** _____

_____ .

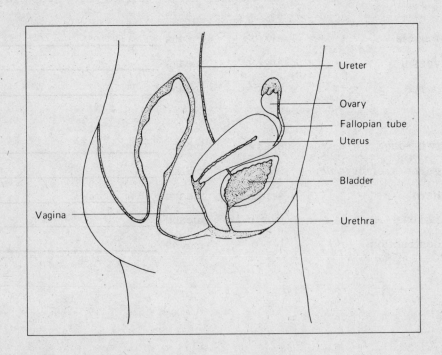

43

An ovum is discharged from the ovary. The
word root-combining form used in words that
refer to the ovary is oophor/o. What does

excision, or surgical
  removal, of the
  ovary

oophor/ectomy mean ? ** _____

_____.

44

Using what you need from oophor/o, build a
word that means:

oophor/itis
oophoritis
o of o ri' tis

inflammation of an ovary,

_____ / _____ ;

oophor/ectomy
oophorectomy
o of o rek' to me

excision of an ovary,

_____ / _____ ;

oophor/oma
oophoroma
o of o ro' ma

tumor of an ovary (ovarian tumor),

_____ / _____ .

45

Oophoropexy means fixation of a displaced
ovary. Pex/o is a word root-combining form

fixation (of)

that means _____ .

46

When an ovary is displaced, a surgical procedure to fix it back in its normal place is called

oophor/o/pex/y
oophoropexy
o of' o ro pek si

_____ / ___ / _____ .

47

The surgical procedure for a prolapsed
(dropped or sagged) ovary is called an

oophoropexy

_____ .

48

Salping/o is used to build words that refer to the fallopian tube(s). A salpingoscope is an instrument used to examine the

fallopian tube(s)   *_____.

49

Using what you need of salping/o, build a word meaning:

salping/itis   inflammation of a fallopian tube,
salpingitis
sal pin ji' tis   _____/_____;

salping/ectomy   excision of a fallopian tube,
salpingectomy
sal pin jek' to me   _____/_____;

salping/ostomy   a surgical opening into a fallopian tube,
salpingostomy
sal pin gos' to me   _____/_____.

50

In words built from laryng/o, pharyng/o, and salping/o, the "g" is pronounced as a hard "g" when followed by an "o" or an "a." The "g" in good is a hard "g"; for example, in laryngalgia and salpingocele, the "g" of the word root is

game and good   pronounced hard as in _____.
  (pronounce them)   (game/good/germ/giant)

51

In laryngostomy, pharyngotomy, and salpingo-

hard   pexy, the "g" is given a _____ sound.
  (pronounce them)   (hard/soft)

52

o and a   A hard "g" precedes the vowels _____ and _____.

53

In words built from laryng/o, pharyng/o, and salping/o, the "g" is soft when followed by an "e" or an "i." The "g" in germ and giant is soft; for example in laryngectomy and salping-

germ and giant
  (pronounce them)

itis, the "g" is soft as in _____.
                              (game/good) (germ/giant)

54

In salpingian, laryngitis, and pharyngectomy,

soft
  (pronounce them)

the "g" is given a_____ sound because
                    (soft/hard)

e and i

it precedes the vowels _____ and _____.

55

laryng e ctomy
pharyngalgia
pharyng i tis
salpingo-
  oophorectomy

Circle the vowels in each of the following words that mean that the "g" is given the soft "j" sound:

laryngectomy   pharyngitis

pharyngalgia   salpingo-oophorectomy

56

salping/o/oophor/
  itis
salpingo-oophor-
  itis
sal ping go-o o for
  i' tis

When building compound medical words, if two like vowels occur between word roots or combining forms, they are separated by a hyphen. Use salpingo-oophorectomy as a model and build a word that means inflammation of the fallopian tube and ovary:

_____ / / _____ / _____.

57

two like vowels join
  word roots or
  combining forms

In compound words a hyphen (-) is used when

** _____

_____.

58

Hyster/o is used to build words about the uterus. A hyster/ectomy is an excision of the

uterus   _____.

59

Write words for the following:

an incision into the uterus,

hysterotomy   _____;

a spasm of the uterus,

hysterospasm   _____;

surgical fixation of the uterus,

hysteropexy   _____.

60

What is the meaning of a hyster/o/salping/o-

excision, or surgical   oophor/ectomy ? ** _____
removal of, the
uterus, fallopian   _____
tubes, and ovaries
                       _____.

hyster/o/salping/   **61**
    o-/oophor/ectomy   Build the word that means excision of the
hysterosalpingo   uterus, fallopian tubes, and ovaries:
oophorectomy
his ter o sal pin go-   _____ / ____ / _____ / ___ -
o o for ek' to mi
                           _____ / _____.

62

Hyster/o/ptosis means prolapse (sagging) of
the uterus. Ptosis (pronounced to' sis) is a
prolapse or
    sagging   word that means _____.

63

When prolapse occurs, a fixation or hysteropexy, is usually done. A hysteropexy would
hyster/o/ptosis   be done to correct or repair the condition
hysteroptosis
his ter op to' sis   known as _____ / ____ / _____.

64

Many organs can prolapse or sag. When the
uterus prolapses, it is called

hysteroptosis

_____.

65

Blephar/o/ptosis means prolapse of an eyelid.
The word root-combining form for eyelid is

blephar/o

_____ / ___.

66

Blephar/edema means swelling of the eyelid.
Build a word that means:

blephar/itis
blepharitis
blef ar i' tis

inflammation of the eyelid,

_____ / _____;

blephar/otomy
blepharotomy
blef ar ot' o mi

incision of the eyelid,

_____ / _____;

blephar/o/plast/y
blepharoplasty
blef' ar o plas ti

surgical repair of the eyelid,

_____ / / _____ / ___;

blephar/o/spasm
blepharospasm
blef' ar o spazm

twitching of the eyelid,

_____ / / _____;

blephar/o/ptosis
blepharoptosis
blef ar op to' sis

prolapse of the eyelid,

_____ / / _____.

67

Nephr/o is used in words to refer to the kidney.
A word that means prolapse of the kidney is

nephr/o/ptosis
nephroptosis
nef rop to' sis

_____ / / _____.

Build a word meaning:

nephr/o/pex/y
nephropexy
nef' ro peks i

fixation of a kidney,

_____ / / _____ / ___;

nephr/o/lysis
nephrolysis
nef rol' i sis

destruction of kidney tissue,

_____/___/_____;

nephr/itis
nephritis
nef ri' tis

inflammation of a kidney,

_____/_____;

nephr/o/lith
nephrolith
nef' ro lith

stone in the kidney,

_____/___/_____;

nephr/o/megaly
nephromegaly
nef ro meg' a li

enlargement of the kidney,

_____/___/_____.

68
The urinary tract is responsible for forming
urine from waste materials in the blood and
eliminating urine from the body. What is the

ur   word root for urine? _____.

69
Here is a brief summary of the functions of
each part of the urinary tract:

kidney   - forms urine,
renal pelvis   - collects urine in the kidney,
ureter   - carries urine to the bladder,
bladder   - stores urine until voiding,
urethra   - discharges urine from the body.

On the following page is a chart to help you
work frames 70 to 80. While learning terminology related to the urinary tract refer to this
chart and the summary above.

WORD	WORD-ROOT COMBINING FORM	NEW SUFFIX TO USE WHEN NEEDED*
urine kidney	ur/o nephr/o	orrhaphy (suturing or stitching)
renal pelvis ureter	pyel/o ureter/o	orrhagia (hemorrhage or "bursting forth" of blood)
bladder urethra	cyst/o urethr/o	

*Note: These two involve combining forms starting with orrh that can be used as suffixes. You have now learned three of the four orrh suffixes.

renal pelvis	**70** Pyel/o refers to the * _____ .
pyel/itis pyelitis pi el i' tis	**71** Taking what you need from the combining form for renal pelvis, form words meaning: inflammation of the renal pelvis, _____ / _____ ;
pyel/o/plast/y pyeloplasty pi' el o plas ti	surgical repair of the renal pelvis, _____ / _____ / _____ .
condition of the renal pelvis and kidney	**72** Pyel/o/nephr/osis means ** _____ _____ .
pyel/o/nephr/itis pyelonephritis pi el o nef ri' tis	Form a word that means inflammation of the renal pelvis and kidney: _____ / _____ / _____ .

73

stone or calculus
in the ureter

Ureter/o/lith means ** _____

_____.

Form a word that means incision into the
ureter (for removal of a stone):

ureterolithotomy
or ureterotomy

_____.

74

surgical repair
of the ureter and
renal pelvis

Ureter/o/pyel/o/plast/y means ** _____

_____.

Form a word meaning:

ureter/o/pyel/itis
ureteropyelitis
u re ter o pi el i' tis

inflammation of the ureter and renal pelvis,

_____/_____/_____/_____;

ureter/o/cyst/
ostomy
ureterocystóstomy
u re ter o sis tos'
to mi

making a new opening between the ureter and
bladder,

_____/_____/_____/_____.

75

Ureter/orrhaphy introduces a new word part:
orrhaphy is not really a suffix, but again (for
simplification) it can be used as one; orrhaphy

suturing or stitch-
ing (for the purpose
of correction or
repair)

means ** _____

_____.

76

Form a word meaning:

ureter/orrhaphy
ureterorrhaphy
u re ter or' ra fi

suturing of the ureter,

_____/_____;

nephr/orrhaphy
nephrorrhaphy
nef ror' a fi

suturing of a kidney,

_____/_____;

cyst/orrhaphy
cystorrhaphy
sist or' a fi

suture of the bladder,

_____/_____;

neur/orrhaphy neurorrhaphy nu ror' a fi	suture of a nerve, _____/_____;
blephar/orrhaphy blepharorrhaphy blef a ror' raf i	suturing of the eyelids, _____/_____.

carries urine from
   the body or re-
   moves urine from
   the bladder

77
The urethra is the organ that ** _____

_____.

The word root-combining form for urethra is

urethr/o

_____/___.

78

suturing of
  the urethra

Urethr/orrhaphy means ** _____

_____.

Form a word that means:

urethr/otomy
urethrotomy
u re throt' o mi

incision into the urethra,

_____/_____;

urethr/o/spasm
urethrospasm
u re' thro spazm

spasm of the urethra,

_____/___/_____.

79
Another complex word part is orrhagia, which
can be used as a suffix because it follows a
word root and ends a word; orrhagia means

hemorrhage or
  bursting forth
  of blood

** _____

_____.

80

Build a word that means:

cyst/orrhagia
cystorrhagia
sist or ra' ji a

hemorrhage of the bladder,

_____/_____ ;

ureter/orrhagia
ureterorrhagia
u re ter or ra' ji a

hemorrhage of the ureter,

_____/_____ .

81

Pne/o refers to breathing. The lungs are the organs of the body that take in air (breathe). Pneumon/o is used in medical words concerning lungs. Form a word that means hemorrhage of a lung,

pneumon/orrhagia
pneumonorrhagia
nu mon or ra' ji a

_____/_____ .

82

Pneumon/ia is a disease of the lungs. Virus pneumonia is also called pneumonitis. Therefore two acceptable ways of saying that the patient has a virus infection of lung tissue is to use one word

pneumon/itis
pneumonitis
nu mo' ni' tis

_____/_____

pneumon/ia
pneumonia
nu mo' ni a

or to say virus

_____/_____ .

83

Pneum/o and pneumon/o can both refer to the lungs. Pneum/o is derived from the Greek word pneuma (air). Pneumon/o comes from the Greek word pneumon (lung). When you want to build a word that refers to a lung or the lungs, you may use either

pneum/o

_____/_____ or

pneumon/o

_____/_____ .

84
Your use of pneum/o will be in words about
air. Pneum/o/derm/a means a collection of
air under the skin. A collection of air in the
chest cavity (thorax) is a

pneum/o/thorax
pneumothorax
nu mo tho' raks

_____ / / _____ .

85
Hydrotherapy means treatment with water.
Treatment with compressed air is called

pneum/o/therap/y
pneumotherapy
nu mo ther' a pi

_____ / / _____ / __ .

86
Melan/o means black. Melan/osis means a
condition of black pigmentation. A word that

melan/oma
melanoma
mel an o' ma

means black tumor is _____ / ____ .

melan/o/carcin/
  oma
melanocarcinoma
mel a no kar sin
  o' ma

87
You have already learned that a carcin/oma is
a form of cancer. A darkly pigmented cancer

is _____ / / _____ / ____ .

88
Whenever a hairless mole on the skin turns
black and grows, a physician should be con-
sulted, for there is danger of black-mole

melanocarcinoma

cancer or _____ .

Below are 50 of the medical terms you formed in Unit 4. Pronounce each one aloud before going on to Unit 5.

angioblast	hysteropexy	pneumonitis
angiosclerosis	hysterospasm	pneumotherapy
apnea	hysterotomy	pneumothorax
arteriosclerosis	kinesialgia	pyelitis
arteriospasm	kinesiology	pyeloplasty
blepharoptosis	melanocarcinoma	salpingectomy
blepharorrhaphy	melanoma	salpingo-oophor-
blepharospasm	myosclerosis	ectomy
bradycardia	myospasm	salpingoscopy
bradypnea	nephritis	spermatoblast
cystorrhagia	nephrolith	spermatoid
dysmenorrhea	nephromegaly	tachycardia
dyspepsia	nephroptosis	tachypnea
dyspnea	neurofibroma	ureterolithotomy
hemangiitis	neurolysis	ureterorrhaphy
hematologist	oophorectomy	ureterotomy
hemolysis	oophoropexy	urethrotomy

Complete the Unit 4 Self-Test before going on.

UNIT 4   SELF-TEST

From the list on the right select the correct meaning for each of the following terms:

_____ 1. Blepharospasm

_____ 2. Spermatoid

_____ 3. Nephroptosis

_____ 4. Melanoma

_____ 5. Oophoropexy

_____ 6. Bradypnea

_____ 7. Angioblast

_____ 8. Ureterotomy

_____ 9. Angiosclerosis

_____ 10. Hysterotomy

_____ 11. Myospasm

_____ 12. Dyspepsia

_____ 13. Hemolysis

_____ 14. Kinesiology

_____ 15. Pneumotherapy

a. The study (or science of) motion

b. A condition of hardening of vessels

c. Twitching of the eyelid

d. Destruction of blood (cells)

e. Abnormally slow breathing

f. Surgical fixation of the ovary

g. Tumor of nerve and fibrous tissue

h. Muscle spasm ("charlie horse")

i. Black tumor

j. Resembling sperm

k. Abnormally enlarged kidney

l. Treatment using air

m. Painful menstruation (cramps)

n. Embryonic vessel cell

o. Kidney out of its normal place (dropped kidney)

p. Incision into the uterus (cesarean section)

q. Painful digestion ("heartburn")

r. Incision into the ureter

PART 2

Complete each of the medical terms on the right with the appropriate missing part:

1. A condition of hardening of muscle   _____ sclerosis

2. Kidney stone   Nephro _____

3. Abnormally fast breathing   Tachy _____

4. Painful menstruation   _____ menorrhea

5. Spasm of the uterus   _____ spasm

6. Cessation of breathing   _____ pnea

7. Hemorrhage (bleeding) from the bladder   _____ orrhagia

8. Surgical removal of the ovary   _____ ectomy

9. Incision into the ureter (for the purpose of removing a stone)   _____ lithotomy

10. Surgical removal of the fallopian tube   _____ ectomy

11. Air in the chest cavity   Pneumo _____

12. Muscle pain due to motion   _____ algia

13. Spasm of the vessels   _____ spasm

14. Inflammation of the lungs (another word for pneumonia)   Pneumon _____

15. Incision into the urethra   _____ otomy

ANSWERS

Part 1

1. c	9. b
2. j	10. p
3. o	11. h
4. i	12. q
5. f	13. d
6. e	14. a
7. n	15. l
8. r	

Part 2

1. Myosclerosis
2. Nephrolith
3. Tachypnea
4. Dysmenorrhea
5. Hysterospasm
6. Apnea
7. Cystorrhagia
8. Oophorectomy

9. Ureterolithotomy
10. Salpingectomy
11. Pneumothorax
12. Kinesialgia
13. Angiospasm
14. Pneumonitis
15. Urethrotomy

Unit 5

In this unit you will make more than 150 new medical terms. Some
words will be formed by using parts you already know. You will also
use the following new word root-combining forms, prefixes, and
suffixes:

algesia (abnormal sensitivity)
cheil/o (lip)
col/o (colon)
dactyl/o (fingers or toes)
dipl/o (two, double)
drom/o (running with, symptom)
ectasia (dilatation, stretching)
enter/o (intestine)
esophag/o (esophagus)
esthesia (feeling)
gingiv/o (gums)
gloss/o (tongue)
hepat/o (liver)

ile/o (ileum)
jejun/o (jejunum)
myel/o (spinal cord, bone marrow)
pancreat/o (pancreas)
phas/o (speech)
phleb/o (veins)
plas/o (formation)
proct/o (rectum and anus)
psych/o (mind)
rect/o (rectum)
stomat/o (mouth)
therm/o (heat)

dia- (through)
macro- (large)
micro- (small)
poly- (many)
pro- (before)
syn- (together)

-clysis (irrigation)
-ectasia (dilation)
-gnosis (know)
-opia (vision)
-orrhexis (rupture)
-plegia, plegic (paralysis)
-tripsy (crushing)

1

Refer to the following illustration and chart to work through frame 32. Food passes through the digestive system in the order of the organs listed in the chart (except for the gallbladder and the appendix).

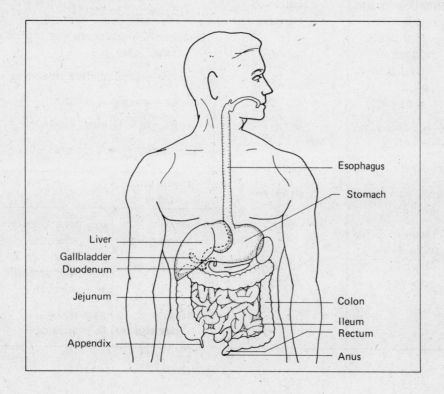

ORGAN	WORD ROOT COMBINING FORM FOR ORGAN	ANOTHER WORD ROOT OR COMBINING FORM	
mouth	stomat/o	algia – pain	
teeth	dent/o	clysis – washing or irrigation (word in itself)	
tongue	gloss/o		
lips	cheil/o		
gums	gingiv/o	plasty – surgical repair (plastic surgery)	
esophagus	esophag/o	cele – herniation	
stomach	gastr/o		
small intestine	enter/o	ectasia – dilatation or stretching (word in itself)	
duodenum (1st part)	duoden/o	centesis – puncture (or tap) to draw fluid	
jejunum (2nd part)	jejun/o		
ileum (3rd part)	ile/o	ptosis – prolapse or drooping	
		pexy – surgical fixation	
large intestine or colon	col/o	orrhagia – hemorrhage	
		orrhaphy – suturing of	
rectum	rect/o		
anus and rectum	proct/o	combining form	suffix
glands of digestion		scop/o (examine)	e – noun (instrument)
liver	hepat/o		y – noun (process or action)
pancreas	pancreat/o		ic – adjective
		pleg/a (paralysis)	ia – noun
			ic – adjective

2
The word root-combining form for mouth is

stomat/o   _____ / __ .

3

inflammation of
the mouth

Stomat/itis means ** _____

_____.

surgical repair
of the mouth

Stomat/o/plast/y means ** _____

_____.

4

Using the word root for mouth, form a word
meaning:

stomat/algia
stomatalgia
sto mat al' ji a

pain in the mouth,

_____ / _____ ;

stomat/orrhagia
stomatorrhagia
sto ma tor ra' ji a

hemorrhage of the mouth,

_____ / _____.

5

Refer to the chart. The word root-combining

gloss/o

form for tongue is _____ / _____ .

Gloss/algia means ** _____

pain in the tongue

_____.

excision of
the tongue

Gloss/ectomy means ** _____

_____.

spasm or twitch-
ing of the tongue

Gloss/o/spasm means ** _____

_____.

6

Using the word root, build a word meaning:

gloss/itis
glossitis
glos si' tis

inflammation of the tongue,

_____ / _____ ;

gloss/al
glossal
glos' sal

pertaining to the tongue,

_____ / al .

7

hypo/gloss/al
hypoglossal
hi po glos' sal

What word would you use to describe a medication that is administered under the tongue ?

_____/_____/_____ medication.

8

Using the information needed from the chart, build a word meaning:

gloss/o/pleg/ia
glossoplegia
glos so ple' ji a

paralysis of the tongue (noun),

_____/ /_____/_____;

gloss/o/pleg/ic
glossoplegic
glos so ple' jic

paralysis of the tongue (adjective),

_____/ /_____/_____.

9

Go back to the chart. The word root for lip is

cheil

_____. The combining form for lip is

cheil/o

_____/__.

10

inflammation
of the lips

Cheil/itis means ** _____

_____.

plastic surgery
of the lips

Cheil/o/plast/y means ** _____

_____.

11

Build a word meaning:

cheil/otomy
cheilotomy
ki lot' o mi

incision of the lips,

_____/_____;

cheil/osis
cheilosis
ki lo' sis

abnormal condition or morbid condition of the

lips, _____/_____.

cheil/o/stomat/o/
  plast/y
cheilostomatoplasty
ki lo sto mat' o
  plas te

12
A word meaning plastic surgery of the lips
and mouth is

_____ / / _____ / / _____ / .
  lip   mouth   repair suffix

13
The word root-combining form for gums is

gingiv/o   _____ / ___.   Gingival means

pertaining to gums   ** _____.

14
Build a word meaning:

gingiv/itis
gingivitis   inflammation of the gums,
jin ji vi' tis
                        _____ / _____ ;

gingiv/algia
gingivalgia   gum pain,
jin ji val' ji a
                        _____ / _____ ;

gingiv/ectomy
gingivectomy   excision of gum tissue,
jin ji vek' to mi
                        _____ / _____ ;

gingiv/o/gloss/itis
gingivoglossitis   inflammation of the gums and tongue,
jin ji vo glos si' tis
                        _____ / / _____ / _____ .

15
Here are some easy ones.

stomach   Gastr/orrhagia means ** _____
  hemorrhage
                        _____ .

inflammation   Gastr/itis means ** _____
  of the stomach
                        _____ .

pertaining to   Gastr/ic means ** _____
  the stomach
                        _____ .

16
Go back to the chart for help on this one. Form a word meaning:

gastr/ectasia
gastrectasia
gas trec' ta si a

dilatation (stretching) of the stomach,

_____/_____ ;

gastr/o/enter/
  ostomy
gastroenterostomy
gas tro en ter os'
  to me

surgical procedure to form a new opening between the stomach and small intestine,

_____/ /_____/_____ ;

gastr/o/enter/ic
gastroenteric
gas tro en ter' ic

pertaining to the stomach and small intestine,

_____/ /_____/____ .

17
Refer to the chart again. Build a word meaning:

enter/o/clysis
enteroclysis
en ter ok' li sis

washing or irrigation of the small intestine,

_____/ /_____ ;

enter/ectasia
enterectasia
en ter ec ta' si a

dilatation of the small intestine,

_____/_____ .

18
What do the following terms mean?

an instrument to
  examine the
  small intestine

Enter/o/scope ** _____

_____ .

puncture of the
  small intestine

Enter/o/centesis ** _____

_____ .

Enter/o/cele ** _____

intestinal hernia

_____ .

19

Try these.

pertaining to the
colon or large
intestine

Col/ic ** _____

_____.

puncture of
the colon

Col/o/centesis ** _____

_____.

making a new open-
ing into the colon

Col/ostomy ** _____

_____.

20

Build a word meaning:

col/o/pex/y
colopexy
ko' lo pek si

surgical fixation of the colon,

_____ / _____ / _____ ;

col/o/clysis
coloclysis
ko lok' li sis

washing or irrigation of the colon,

_____ / _____ / _____ ;

col/itis
colitis
ko li' tis

inflammation of the colon,

_____ / _____ .

21

Refer to your chart again. The word root-com-

rect/o

bining form for rectum is _____ / _____ .

What do each of the following mean?

pertaining to
the rectum

Rect/al ** _____

_____.

Rect/o/cele ** _____

a rectal hernia

_____.

washing or irriga-
tion of the rectum

Rect/o/clysis ** _____

_____.

22

rect/o/urethr/al
rectourethral
rek to u re' thral

Build a word meaning:

pertaining to the rectum and urethra,

_____ / / _____ / _____;

rect/o/cyst/otomy
rectocystotomy
rek to sis tot' o mi

incision of the bladder through the rectum,

_____ / / _____ / _____.
　　　　　rectum　　　　　bladder　　　　incision

23

specializes in
　diseases of anus
　and rectum

See the chart for help. A proct/o/log/ist is

one who ** _____

_____.

the study of diseases
　of anus and rectum

Proct/o/log/y is ** _____

_____.

24

proct/o/clysis
proctoclysis
prok tok' li sis

proctoplegia or
　proctoparalysis

Build a word meaning:

washing or irrigation of anus and rectum,

_____ / / _____;

paralysis of the opening from the anus,

_____.

25

instrument for
　examining the
　anus and rectum

Write a meaning for each of the following:

proct/o/scope ** _____

_____.

examination of the
　anus and rectum

proct/o/scopy ** _____

_____.

26
Back to the chart.   Hepat/ic means

pertaining to
   the liver

** _____ .

enlargement of
   the liver

Hepatomegaly means ** _____

_____ .

27
Build a word meaning:

hepat/o/scop/y
hepatoscopy
hep a tos' kop e

inspection (examination) of the liver,

_____ / / _____ / ;

hepat/otomy
hepatotomy
hep a tot' o mi

incision into the liver,

_____ / _____ ;

hepat/itis
hepatitis
hep a ti' tis

inflammation of the liver,

_____ / _____ .

28
Another new word root-combining form.

pertaining to
   the pancreas

Pancreat/ic means ** _____

_____ .

destruction of
   pancreatic tissue

Pancreat/o/lys/is means ** _____

_____ .

29
Build a word meaning:

pancreat/o/lith
pancreatolith
pan kre at' o lith

a stone or calculus in the pancreas,

_____ / / _____ ;
       pancreas   stone

pancreat/itis
pancreatitis
pan kre at i' tis

inflammation of the pancreas,

_____ / _____ ;

pancreat/ectomy
pancreatectomy
pan kre at ek' to mi

excision of part or all of the pancreas,

_____ / _____ ;

pancreat/otomy
pancreatotomy
pan kre at ot' o mi

incision into the pancreas,

_____ / _____ .

30
When an entire gastrectomy is performed, a
new connection (opening) is formed between the
esophagus and duodenum. This is called an

esophag/o/duoden/
  ostomy
esophagoduoden-
  ostomy
e sof a go du o den
  os' to me

_____ / / _____ / _____ .

(Note: Remember to name the anatomical parts
in the order in which food passes through them.)

31
As you rewrite each of the following, analyze
it (make your own diagonal divisions):

gastro/o/enter/o/
  col/ostomy

gastroenterocolostomy,

_____ ;

esophag/o/gastr/
  ostomy

esophagogastrostomy,

_____ ;

enter/o/chol/e/
  cyst/ostomy

enterocholecystostomy,

_____ .

32
Try it again:

jejun/o/ile/
  ostomy

jejunoileostomy,

_____ ;

duoden/o/chol/e/
  cyst/ostomy

duodenocholecystostomy,

_____ ;

esophag/o/gastr/
  o/scopy

esophagogastroscopy,

_____ .

33
Arteries are vessels (angi/o) that carry blood
from the heart. Veins are vessels that carry

heart

blood back to the _____ .

34
A word root-combining form for vein is
phleb/o. Arteriosclerosis is hardening of the

arteries

_____.

phleb/o/scler/osis
phlebosclerosis
fleb o skle ro' sis

Hardening of veins is called

_____/___/_____.
    vein   hardening

35
Build a word meaning:

phleb/otomy
phlebotomy
fleb ot' o mi

incision in a vein (venisection or cut-down),

_____/_____;

phleb/itis
phlebitis
fleb i' tis

inflammation of a vein,

_____/_____.

36
Another combining form that you can use as a
suffix is orrhexis; orrhexis means rupture,

hyster/orrhexis means ** _____

rupture of
  the uterus

_____.

37
With orrhexis you have learned the last of the
"rrh" forms. Neither of the four is a real
suffix, but since they have involved development you are fortunate to be able to use them

suffixes

as _____.

38
Cyst/orrhexis means ** _____

rupture of
  the bladder

_____.

rupture of the
  small intestine

Enter/orrhexis means ** _____

_____.

39

Build a word meaning:

cardi/orrhexis
cardiorrhexis
kar di or reks' is

rupture of the heart,

_____/_____;

phleb/orrhexis
phleborrhexis
fleb or reks' is

rupture of a vein,

_____/_____.

40

Here's a chance to use all the "rrh" forms.
Build a word meaning:

rupture of the bladder,

cyst/orrhexis

_____/_____;

hemorrhage from the liver,

hepat/orrhagia

_____/_____;

flowing from the nose ("running" nose),

rhin/orrhea

_____/_____;

suturing (or joining) the fallopian tubes,

salping/orrhaphy

_____/_____.

suturing (or join-
ing) a rupture

What does herniorrhaphy mean?

**_____.

41

An is a form of the prefix a meaning without.
Esthesia means feeling or sensation. Give
the meaning of the following words:

instrument for
measuring feel-
ing or sensation

esthesiometer ** _____

_____;

abnormal sensi-
tivity (to pain)

hyperesthesia ** _____

_____;

a drug that removes
feeling (literally,
without feeling)

anesthesia ** _____

_____

_____;

the study or science
  of removing feeling

anesthesiolcgy ** _____

_____.

42
Analyze the following words (you do the
dividing):

an/esthesi/o/
  log/ist

anesthesiologist,

_____;

hypoesthesia,

hypo/esthesi/a

_____.

43
If algesia is a word meaning oversensitivity to
pain, what does analgesia mean?

without sensitivity
  to pain

** _____.

44
Write a meaning for each of the following
(phas/o means speech):

speechless

aphasia ** _____;

abnormally
  fast speech

tachyphasia ** _____

_____;

abnormally
  slow speech

bradyphasia ** _____

_____;

pain or difficulty
  when speaking

dysphasia ** _____

_____.

45

My/o is used in words referring to muscle (or muscles). Write a meaning for :

heart muscle

myocardia ** _____ ;

inflammation of heart muscle

myocarditis ** _____

_____ ;

tumor of fibrous tissue and muscle

myofibroma ** _____

_____ .

46

Build a word meaning:

a record or chart of muscle contractions,

my/o/gram

_____ / / _____ ;

an instrument for recording muscle contrac-

my/o/graph

tions, _____ / / _____ ;

the process of recording muscle contractions,

my/o/graph/y

_____ / / _____ / __ .

47

Give a meaning for each of the following:

fatty tumor of the muscle

myolipoma ** _____

_____ ;

resembling muscle

myoid ** _____ ;

the study of the movement of muscle

myokinesiology ** _____

_____ .

48

When you see my/o, you will think of

muscles

_____ .

49

Dipl/o means double or paired; opia is an involved form that we may use as a suffix meaning vision. What does dipl/opia mean?

double vision

**_____.

50

dipl/opia
diplopia
dip lo' pi a

Whenever both eyes fail to record the same image on the brain, a double image occurs.

The medical term is _____ / _____.

51

Give a brief meaning for each of the following:

a family of bacteria
  (coccus) that
  grows in pairs

dipl/o/coccus **_____

_____;

blue vision

cyan/opia **_____.

52

Neur/o is used in words that refer to nerves.

pain along the
  course of a nerve
  (or equivalent)

Neur/algia means **_____

_____.

53

Neurology is the medical speciality that deals with the nervous system. A man who specializes in diseases of the nervous system is a

neur/o/log/ist
neurologist
nu rol' o jist

_____ / _____ / _____ / _____.

54

Build a word meaning:

neur/itis
neuritis
nu ri' tis

inflammation of a nerve, _____ / _____;

neur/o/lysis
neurolysis
nu rol' is is

destruction of nerve tissue,

_____ / _____ / _____;

neur/o/plast/y
neuroplasty
nu' ro plas ti

surgical repair of nerves,

_____ / _____ / _____.

55

Neur/o/trips/y means surgical crushing of a
nerve. The word root for crushing (usually by

trips   rubbing or grinding) is _____.

56

Tripsis, from which we get trips/y, is a Greek
word that means "rub" or "massage." Tripsis
can be carried to the point of crushing or
neur/o/trips/y   grinding. Surgical crushing of a nerve is
neurotripsy
nu' ro trip si   _____ / / _____ / ___.

57

In some cases of lithiasis it may be necessary
to crush calculi so they may be passed. A
word that means surgical crushing of stones is

lith/o/trips/y   _____ / / _____ / ___.

58

Myel/itis can mean either inflammation of
bone marrow or inflammation of the spinal
cord. From the definitions you may conclude
that myel is the word root for

spinal cord   *_____ and

bone marrow   *_____.

59

The word ending o/blast, meaning embryonic
(germ), gives rise to something else. In the
word myel/o/blast, the combining form myel

bone marrow   refers to _____, but in
                                          (bone marrow, spinal cord)
                                  the word myel/o/cele, the combining form

spinal cord   refers to _____.
                                          (bone marrow, spinal cord)

herniation of the
spinal cord

60
What does myelocele mean ?   ** _____

_____.

defective (poor
or abnormal)
formation

61
Plas/ia or plas/is means formation or change
in the sense of molding.   This kind of formation
occurs naturally instead of being done by a
plastic surgeon.   Dys/plas/ia means

** _____.

hyper/plas/ia
hyperplasia
hi per pla' zi a

62
A/plas/ia means failure of an organ to develop
properly.   A word that means overgrowth or
too much development is

_____ / _____ / _____.

hypo/plas/ia
hypoplasia
hi po pla' zi a

63
If overdevelopment is hyperplasia, underdevel-
opment is expressed as

_____ / _____ / _____.

64
Using myel/o/dys/plas/ia as a model, build a
word meaning:

chondr/o/dys/
plas/ia

defective development of cartilage,

_____ / ___ / _____ / _____ / ___ ;

oste/o/chondr/o/
dys/plas/ia

defective formation of bone and cartilage,

_____ / ___ / _____ / ___ / _____ / ___.

the soul, the
mind, the
mental life

65
Psych/o comes from the Greek psyche. Look
up psycho and Psyche in a Webster's Collegiate
Dictionary. Give at least one meaning:

** _____.

66

Psychiatry is the field of medicine that studies and deals with mental and neurotic disorders. The physician who specializes in this field of medicine is called a _____.

psychiatrist
si ki' a trist

67

Psych/o/log/y is the science that studies the mind and mental process. The scientist who works in this field is called a

psych/o/log/ist
psychologist
si kol' o gist

_____ / / / _____.

(Psychiatry is the medical branch of psychology.)

68

Psych/o/genesis means the formation or development of mental traits. A word that means any abnormal mental condition is

psych/osis
psychosis
si ko' sis

_____ / _____.

69

A psych/o/neur/osis is a disease that is mainly mental in origin. A psych/o/neur/o/tic person is one who suffers from a

psych/o/neur/osis
psychoneurosis
si ko nu ro' sis

_____ / / / _____.

70

The patient suffering from a psychoneurosis can tell what is real from the unreal. He only exaggerates the reality. What is the adjective that describes a person with a psychoneurosis?

psych/o/neur/o/tic

_____ / / / / _____.

71

Psychoneuroses (plural) take many forms. Hysteria, psych/asthenia, and neur/asthenia

psych/o/neur/oses

are forms of _____ / / / _____.

72

In Webster's dictionary look at the words beginning with gnos. They come from the Greek

knowledge

word <u>gnosis</u>, meaning _____.

73

The prefix pro means before or in front. What do you think is the meaning of pro/gnos/is ?

knowledge that
  comes before; fore-
  knowledge or predic-
  tion of the outcome
  of a disease

** _____

_____

_____.

74

Acute leukemia is usually fatal within three months. Prediction of the outcome of any dis-

pro/gnos/is
prognosis
prog no' sis

ease is called a _____ / _____ / _____.

75

What word means giving an indication to the outcome of a disease ?

pro/gnos/ticate
prognosticate
prog nos' ti kate

_____ / _____ / ticate .
        (verb)

76

Di/a means through. Diagnosis means

know through

literally ** _____.

77

A diagnosis of a disease is made by studying through its symptoms. When a patient tells a physician that he has chills, hot spells, and a runny nose, the physician may make a

di/a/gnos/is
diagnosis
di ag no' sis

_____ / _____ / _____ / __ of a head cold.

78

flowing through
  or running
  through

The literal meaning of di/a/rrhea is

** _____.

79

Di/a/therm/y means generating heat through

through

(tissues). Di/a means _____.

heat

Therm means _____. Y is a noun

suffix or ending

_____.

80

therm/o/meter
thermometer
ther mom' e ter

Therm/o is the word root-combining form
which means heat. An instrument to measure

heat is a _____ / / _____.

81

therm/al or
    therm/ic

Build a word meaning:

pertaining to heat, _____ / ____;

therm/o/algesia
  or therm/o/
  esthesia

oversensitivity to heat,

_____ / / _____;

heating through tissue,

di/a/therm/y

_____ / / _____ / ___.

82

therm or
  therm/o
  (Try it!)

If you ever wanted information about temperature scales or variations of body temperature,
you would look in the dictionary for words be-

ginning with _____.

83

di/a/scop/e
diascope
di' as kop

A micr/o/scop/e is an instrument for examining (or looking at) something small. An instrument for examining, or looking "through," is a

_____ / / _____ / ___.

84

di/a

A diascope is placed on the skin, and the skin
is looked "through" to see changes. The word

part for through is _____ / ___.

micr/o/meter
micrometer
mi krom' e ter

85
An instrument for measuring something micro-

scopic is a _____ / / _____.
The micron (1/1000 mm) is the unit of measurement. Many cocci are 2 microns in diameter.

microns
mi' krons

A red blood cell is 7 _____ in diameter.

86
Macr/o is the opposite of micr/o. Macr/o is

large

used in words to mean _____.

87
Things that are macr/o/scop/ic can be seen
with the naked eye. Give a meaning for

a large embryonic
  (or germ) cell

macroblast. ** _____

_____.

88
An abnormally large head is

macr/o/cephal/us

_____ / / _____ / ____.

An abnormally large cell is a

macr/o/cyte

_____ / / _____.

A very large coccus is called a

macr/o/cocc/us

_____ / / _____ / ____.

89
Macr/o/gloss/ia means ** _____

abnormally
  large tongue

_____.

abnormally
  large ear(s)

Macr/ot/ia means ** _____

_____.

abnormally
  large nose

Macr/o/rhin/ia means ** _____

_____.

abnormally
  large lips

Macr/o/cheil/ia means ** _____

_____.

90

Macr/o/dactyl/ia means abnormally large fingers or toes. The word root for fingers or

dactyl   toes is _____.

91

What does dactyl/o/megal/y mean?

another way of   ** _____
 saying large fin-
 gers or toes   _____.

92

A finger or toe is called a digit. The word

dactyl/o   root-combining form is _____ /____.

                                Build a word meaning:

dactyl/itis   inflammation of a digit,
dactylitis
dak til i' tis   _____ / _____;

dactyl/o/spasm   cramp or spasm of a digit,
dactylospasm
dak' til o spazm   _____ / ____ / _____;

dactyl/o/gram   a fingerprint,
dactylogram
dak til' o gram   _____ / ____ / _____.

abnormally large   **93**
 fingers and toes   Macr/o/dactyl/ia means ** _____
 (digits)
                                _____.

fingers or toes   Poly/dactyl/ism means too many ** _____
 (digits)
                                _____.

94

Pol/y is a combining form that means too many
or too much. Pol/y/ur/ia means excessive
pol/y/ur/ia   amount of urine. When a person drinks too
polyuria
pol i u' ri a   much water, _____ / __ / ___ / _____ results.

95

pol/y/neur/itis
polyneuritis
pol i nu ri' tis

Pol/y/neur/o/path/y means disease of many nerves. The word for inflammation of many

nerves is _____/___/_____/_____.

96

Build a word meaning:

pol/y/arthr/itis
polyarthritis
pol i ar thri' tis

inflammation of many joints,

_____/___/_____/_____;

pol/y/neur/algia
polyneuralgia
pol i nu ral' ji a

pain in several nerves,

_____/___/_____/_____.

97

syn/ergetic
synergetic
sin er jet' ik

Syn/ergetic means working together. Drugs that work together to increase one another's

effect are called _____/_____ drugs.

98

synergetic

Synergetic muscles are muscles that work to-gether. There are three muscles that work together to flex the forearm. They are

_____ muscles.

99

synergetic

APC tablets are more effective for killing pain than aspirin alone. This is because aspirin, phenacetin, and caffeine are

_____ drugs.

100

joining of two
   or more digits

What does syn/dactyl/ism mean (ism is a noun

suffix) ? ** _____

_____.

101

Syn/arthr/osis means an immovable joint; ad-
joining bones are fused together. When bones
are fused at a joint so that there is no movement, the condition is called

syn/arthr/osis
synarthrosis
sin ar thro' sis

_____/_____/_____.

102

A syn/drome is a variety of symptoms occurring (meaning running along) together. The
complete picture of a disease is its

syn/drome
syndrome
sin' drom

_____/_____.

103

Alcoholism produces a characteristic group of
symptoms called Korsakoff's syndrome. From
the name we know that a variety of symptoms

together   occurs _____.

104

Pro/drome means running before (a disease).
Symptoms that indicate an approaching disease

pro/drome
prodrome
pro' drom   are its _____/_____.

105

The sneezes that come before a common cold

prodrome   are the _____ of the cold.

106

A rash that shows before the true macules of
measles are evident is described as a

pro/drom/al
prodromal
prod' ro mal   _____/_____/_____ rash.
                   (adjective ending)

In this unit you worked with more than 150 new medical terms. Fifty of those words are listed here for you to practice your pronunciation. Do that first; then take the Unit 5 Self-Test.

analgesia	gingivoglossitis	micrometer
anesthesiologist	glossoplegia	myeloblast
cardiorrhexis	gastrectasia	myokinesiology
cheilitis	gastrorrhagia	neuromyelitis
cheiloplasty	hepatitis	neurotripsy
colic	hepatomegaly	pancreatectomy
colitis	hepatorrhagia	phlebitis
colostomy	herniorrhaphy	polyarthritis
cystorrhexis	hyperesthesia	polyuria
dactylogram	hypoesthesia	psychoneurosis
dactylomegaly	hypoglossal	proctoclysis
diathermy	hysterorrhexis	proctoscopy
diplopia	ileoplegia	prognosis
enterocele	jejunoileostomy	rectal
enteroclysis	lithotripsy	syndactylism
esophagogastroscopy	macrocephalus	syndrome
esthesiometer	macrocheilia	

UNIT 5   SELF-TEST

PART 1

From the list on the right, select the correct meaning for each of the following often used medical terms.

_____ 1. Lithotripsy

_____ 2. Proctoclysis

_____ 3. Polyarthritis

_____ 4. Diplopia

_____ 5. Colic

_____ 6. Phlebitis

_____ 7. Glossoplegia

_____ 8. Dactylogram

_____ 9. Analgesia

_____ 10. Cheilitis

_____ 11. Neuromyelitis

_____ 12. Macrocephalus

_____ 13. Hypoesthesia

_____ 14. Hepatomegaly

_____ 15. Syndrome

a. Inflammation of the vein

b. Abnormal enlargement of the liver

c. Washing or irrigation of the small intestine

d. Crushing (destruction) of a nerve

e. Paralysis of the tongue

f. Abnormally enlarged head

g. Absence of pain

h. Inflammation of many joints

i. Under the tongue (sublingual)

j. Double vision

k. Crushing of a calculus

l. Relating to the colon

m. Fingerprint

n. Symptoms that occur together

o. Measurement of feeling or sensation

p. Irrigation of the rectum and anal canal (enema)

q. Inflammation of the nerves of the spinal cord

r. Less than normal sensation

s. Inflammation of the lips

PART 2

Complete each of the medical terms on the right with the appropriate missing part. Some terms are missing all parts!

1. Rupture of the bladder _____ orrhexis

2. Abnormally intense feeling or
    sensation (pain) _____ esthesia

3. Knowing before hand or pre-
    dicting the outcome _____ gnosis

4. Rupture of the uterus Hyster _____

5. Abnormally enlarged lips Macro _____

6. Stretching or dilatation of the
    stomach _____ ectasia

7. Paralysis of the ileum Ileo _____

8. Heat that goes through _____ thermy

9. Abnormally enlarged fingers Dactylo _____

10. Inflammation of the liver _____

11. Instrument for measuring
     sensation _____ meter

12. Relating to the rectum _____

13. Formation of a new opening in
     the colon _____

14. Study of muscle movement _____ kinesi _____

15. Growing together of fingers
     and toes Syn _____ ism

ANSWERS

Part 1

1. k	9. g
2. p	10. s
3. h	11. q
4. j	12. f
5. l	13. r
6. a	14. b
7. e	15. n
8. m	

Part 2

1. Cystorrhexis
2. Hyperesthesia
3. Prognosis
4. Hysterorrhexis
5. Macrocheilia
6. Gastrectasia
7. Ileoplegia
8. Diathermy
9. Dactylomegaly
10. Hepatitis
11. Esthesiometer
12. Rectal
13. Colostomy
14. Myokinesiology
15. Syndactylism

Unit 6

In Unit 6 you will put together more than 60 new medical terms. You will use some of the terms and parts you have already covered and also the following:

anter/o (before, in front of)
caud/o (tail)
chlor/o (green)
dors/o (back)
erythr/o (red)
gynec/o (women)
hidr/o (sweat)
lapar/o (abdominal wall)
later/o (side)

-stasis (slow, stop)
-emia (blood)

men/o (menses)
ophthalm/o (eye)
poster/o (behind)
pyr/o (fire, fever)
syphil/o (syphilis)
ventr/o (belly)
viscer/o (gut, content of abdomen)
xanth/o (yellow)

In the biological sciences there are many directional words. This page is to help you understand the use of six of them. Label the drawings below on the basis of the information given in the chart. Use this page while working frame 1.

DIRECTIONAL WORD	COMBINING FORM	MEANING
dorsal	dors/al – dors/o (back)	near or on the back
ventral	ventr/al – ventr/o (belly)	near or on the belly side of the body
anterior	anter/ior – anter/o (before)	toward the front or in front of
posterior	poster/ior – poster/o (behind, after)	following or located behind
cephalic	cephal/ic – cephal/o (head)	upward – toward the head
caudal caudad	caud/al – caud/o /ad (tail)	downward – toward the tail

Dog   Man

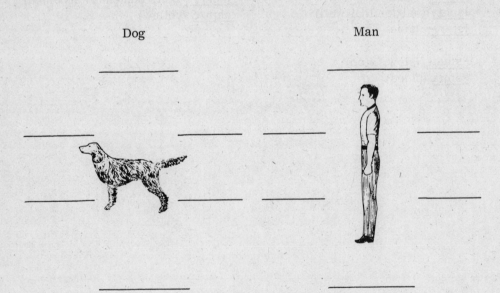

Check your answers with the correct labels on the next page.

1

What is the direction indicated by each of the following:

toward the front
and side

anterolateral ** _____ ;
(side)

toward the front
and middle

anteromedian ** _____ ;
(middle)

toward the front
and above

anterosuperior ** _____ ;
(above)

toward the back
and side

posterolateral ** _____ ;
(side)

Dog	Man

dorsal   _cephalic_

anterior   _posterior_   _ventral_   _dorsal_

cephalic   _caudad (al)_ _anterior_   _posterior_

ventral   _caudad (al)_

2

Men/o is used in words referring to the menses. Men/ses is another way of saying men/struation. Men/o in any word should

menses or
  menstruation

make you think of _____ .

3

menstruation
or menses

Men/o/pause (a normal physiological happening between age 38–50) means permanent cessation of _____.

Men/orrhagia means ** _____

excessive menstrua-
tion or menstrual
hemorrhage

_____

_____.

4

men/orrhea
menorrhea
men or e' a

Build a word meaning:

flow of menses, _____/_____;

dys/men/orrhea
dysmenorrhea
dis men or e' a

painful (bad or difficult) menstrual flow,

_____/_____/_____;

a/men/orrhea
amenorrhea
a men o re' a

absence (without) menstrual flow,

____/_____/_____.

5

controlling
blood flow

Stasis is a word meaning stopping, slowing, or controlling. Hem/o/stasis means

** _____.

phleb/o/stasis
phlebostasis
fleb os' ta sis
(also venostasis)

A word meaning slowing of flow in veins is

_____/___/_____.

6

Syphilis is a veneral disease. Read about the disease in your dictionary. Note the origin of the word. Look at the words beginning with syphil. The combining form used in words re-

syphil/o

ferring to this disease is _____/___.

7

Build a word meaning:

a syphilitic tumor,

syphil/oma   _____/_____;

resembling syphilis,

syphil/oid   _____/_____.

8

The viscera are the internal organs of the body. The word root-combining form for viscera is

viscer/o   _____/_____.

9

Build a word meaning:

viscer/o/ptosis
visceroptosis   prolapse of organs,
vis er op to' sis

_____/_____/_____;

viscer/algia
visceralgia   pain in organs,
vis er al' ji a

_____/_____;

viscer/al
visceral   pertaining to organs,
vis' ser al

_____/_____.

10

Lapar/o means abdominal wall. A laparectomy is an excision of part of the

abdominal wall   *_____.

11

lapar/otomy
laparotomy   Write a word for an incision into the abdominal
lap ar ot' o mi   wall: _____/_____.

lapar/orrhaphy
laparorrhaphy   A suturing of the abdominal wall is
lap ar or' ra fi

_____/_____.

12

lapar/o/hyster/
o/salping/o-
/oophor/ectomy
You couldn't be
wrong!

There may be longer words than this. If there
are, there are not many. Analyze it for fun.
Think of the word parts:
laparohysterosalpingo-oophorectomy

_____

_____.

13

fires

Pyr/o is used in words to mean heat or fever.
(Remember the funeral pyres on which the
Greeks and Romans burned their dead?) A
pyromaniac is one who has a madness for

starting or watching _____.

14

pyr/osis
pyrosis
pi ro' sis

Pyr/exia means fever. A condition of heat

(heartburn) is _____/_____.

15

fever or high
    body temperature

A pyr/o/toxin is a toxin (poison) produced by

** _____.

16

Use this information for building words involving color (frames 18 through 23):

leuk/o	white
melan/o	black
erythr/o	red
cyan/o	blue
chlor/o	green
xanth/o	yellow

17
Cyan/opia means blue vision.   Form a word meaning:

xanth/opia
xanthopia
zan thop' i a   yellow vision, _____/_____;

chlor/opia
chloropia
klo ro' pi a   green vision, _____/_____.

18
Cyan/o/derma means blue skin.   Build a word meaning

red skin (blushing),

erythr/o/derma   _____/ /_____;

black (discolored) skin,

melan/o/derma   _____.
(You pronounce them.) (You draw the lines.)

19
Build a word meaning:

green cell (plants only),

chlor/o/cyte   _____/ /_____;

white (blood) cell,

leuk/o/cyte   _____/ /_____;

red (blood) cell,

erythr/o/cyte   _____/ /_____.
(You pronounce them.)

20
Build a word meaning an embryonic cell of the following color:

melan/o/blast   black, _____/ /_____;

erythr/o/blast   red, _____/ /_____.
(You pronounce them.)

21

Cyan/emia is blue blood (not literally in people; lobsters have blue blood). Build words involving the following colors in blood:

xanth/emia   yellow _____/_____;

erythr/emia   red (blushing) _____/_____.
(You pronounce them.)

22

green   Chlor/o   means _____.

yellow   Xanth/o   means _____.

red   Erythr/o   means _____.

white   Leuk/o   means _____.

black   Melan/o   means _____.

23

Hydr/o means water or fluid. Hidr/o means sweat. A hidr/o/cyst/oma is a cystic tumor of

sweat   a _____ gland.

24

Both hydr/o and hidr/o are pronounced alike.

water or fluid   Hydro with a "y" means _____.

sweat   Hidro with an "i" means _____.

25

inflammation of   Hidr/o/aden/itis means ** _____
  sweat glands   _____.

26

There are three words that mean excessive sweating. Analyze them:

hidr/osis   hidrosis, _____;

hyper/hidr/osis   hyperhidrosis, _____;

hidr/orrhea   hidrorrhea, _____.
(You pronounce them.)

without sweat
  or absence
  of sweat

27
The word an/hidr/osis means ** _____

_____ .

28
Gynec/o comes from the Greek word <u>gyne</u>,
which means woman. The field of medicine
called gynecology deals with diseases of

women
                _____ .

29
Gynec/o/log/ic or gynec/o/log/ical are adjectival forms of gynecology. The physician who
specializes in female disorders is called a

gynec/o/log/ist
gynecologist
jin e kol' o jist

_____ / _____ / _____ / _____ .

30
Ophthalm/o is used in words to mean eye.

inflammation
  of the eye

Ophthalm/itis means ** _____

_____ .

pertaining to
  the eye

Ophthalm/ic means ** _____

_____ .

pain in the
  eye

Ophthalm/algia means ** _____

_____ .

31
Before building words with this root, be sure
you have the phth order of ophthalm/o straight.
Pronounce it off thalm o.

practice pronounc-
  ing the ph th

32

ophthalm/o/cele
ophthalmocele
of thal' mo sel

ophthalm/o/meter
ophthalmometer
of thal mom' et er

opthalm/o/pleg/ia
ophthalmoplegia
of thal mo ple' ji a

Build a word meaning:

herniation of an eye (abnormal protrusion),

_____/ / _____ ;

instrument for measuring the eye,

_____/ / _____ ;

paralysis of the eye,

_____/ / _____/ ____ .

33

ophthalm/o/log/ist

Ophthalmology is the medical speciality of deal-
ing with eye disease. We call the physician who
practices this speciality an

_____/ / _____/ _____ .

34

ophthalm/o/scope

Ophthalm/o/scop/y is the examination of the
interior of the eye. The instrument used for
this examination is an

_____/ / _____ .

35

Fill in the following chart. Check your answers. You will be formally introduced to
some of the specialities in the field of medicine.

SPECIALTY	SPECIALIST	LIMITS OF FIELD
Pathology		Diseases – nature and causes
	Dermatologist	
Neurology		Nervous conditions and diseases
	Gynecologist	
Urology		Urinary diseases and urogenital organs
	Endocrinologist	
Oncology		Neoplasms (new growths)
		Heart
Ophthalmology		Eye
	Otorhinolaryngologist	
Obstetrics		Pregnancy, childbirth, and puerperium
	Geriatrician	Old age
Pediatrics		Children
Orthopedics	Orthopedist	Bones and muscles
Psychiatry		Mental disorders

Check your answers in the next chart.

SPECIALTY	SPECIALIST	LIMITS OF FIELD
	pathologist	
dermatology		skin
	neurologist	
gynecology		
	urologist	
endocrinology		
	oncologist	
cardiology	cardiologist	
	ophthalmologist	
otorhinolaryngology		ear-nose-throat
	obstetrician	
geriatrics		
	pediatrician	
	psychiatrist	

In this unit you formed more than 60 new words. Fifty of these terms are listed to allow you to practice your pronunciation. Pronounce each term several times before you take the Unit 6 Self-Test.

anhidrosis	hidrorrhea	posterior
anterior	hidrosis	posterolateral
anteromedian	hyperhidrosis	psychiatrist
amenorrhea	laparorrhaphy	pyrexia
caudal	laparotomy	pyrotoxin
chlorocyte	leukocyte	syphilis
chloropia	leukemia	syphilitic
dorsal	melanoderma	syphiloid
endocrinology	menopause	syphiloma
erythroblast	menorrhagia	urologist
erythrocyte	menses	venostasis
erythroderma	ophthalmology	ventral
erythremia	ophthalmic	visceral
gynecologist	ophthalmocele	visceralgia
hemostasis	ophthalmoplasty	xanthemia
hidroadenitis	ophthalmoscope	xanthopia
hidrocystoma	phlebostasis	

UNIT 6   SELF-TEST

From the list on the right select the correct meaning for each of the following often-used medical terms:

_____ 1. Pyrexia

_____ 2. Venostasis

_____ 3. Psychiatrist

_____ 4. Erythremia

_____ 5. Hidroadenitis

_____ 6. Caudal

_____ 7. Anterior

_____ 8. Syphiloid

_____ 9. Xanthopia

_____ 10. Chlorocyte

_____ 11. Ophthalmalgia

_____ 12. Menses

_____ 13. Laparorrhaphy

_____ 14. Visceralgia

_____ 15. Leukemia

a. Location in front of

b. Pain in the eye

c. Inflammation of a sweat gland

d. Fever

e. A practitioner who specializes in diseases of the urinary tract

f. Green color of the eye

g. Monthly cycle known as men-struation

h. Slowness of flowing in a vein

i. Painful gut

j. A practitioner who specializes in diseases of the mind

k. Relating to the tail

l. Disease of too many white cells in the blood

m. Abnormal sweating

n. Suturing of the abdominal wall

o. Disease of too many red cells in the blood

p. Yellow color of the eye

q. Resembling syphilis

r. A red blood cell

s. Green color in the cell

PART 2

Complete each of the medical terms on the right with the appropriate missing part. Some terms are missing all parts.

1. A white blood cell   _____cyte

2. Relating to syphilis   _____

3. Relating to the back   _____al

4. Cessation of menses   _____

5. Incision into the abdominal wall   _____otomy

6. A condition of excessive sweating   _____ hidr _____

7. An instrument used for looking
   into the eye   _____ scope

8. Lack of menstrual flow   _____ orrhea

9. Location indicating behind and to
   the side   _____ lateral

10. Yellow color in the blood   Xanth _____

11. Black color of the skin   _____

12. Relating to the front   _____al

13. Red cell   _____

14. Pertaining to the eye   Ophthalm _____

15. Relating to the gut (contents of
    the abdomen)   _____

ANSWERS

Part 1

1. d		9. p
2. h		10. s
3. j		11. b
4. o		12. g
5. c		13. n
6. k		14. i
7. a		15. l
8. q		

Part 2

1. Leukocyte
2. Syphilitic
3. Dorsal
4. Menopause
5. Laparotomy
6. Hyperhidrosis
7. Ophthalmoscope
8. Amenorrhea
9. Dorsolateral or Posterolateral
10. Xanthemia
11. Melanoderma
12. Ventral
13. Erythrocyte
14. Ophthalmic
15. Visceral

Unit 7

In this unit you will form more than 60 medical terms. Some of the new combining forms and prefixes you will use are listed below.

colp/o (vagina)
crypt/o (hidden)
ect/o (outer side)
ectopic (misplaced)
end/o (inner side)
glyc/o (glucose)
heter/o (different)
hom/o (same)
leps/o (seizure)

mes/o (middle)
narc/o (sleep)
necr/o (dead)
orchid/o (testicle)
par/o (bear)
phil/o (attraction)
retr/o (behind, in back of)
splen/o (spleen)

ab- (away from)
auto- (self)
circum- (around)
de- (down from)
ex- (out from)
iso- (equal)
mono- (one)

multi- (many)
nulli- (none)
para- (around, near)
per- (through)
peri- (around)
super- (beyond)
supra- (above)
syn- (together)

1
The cells of the body use a simple sugar, glucose, to release energy. Glyc/o/gen is "animal starch" formed from simple sugars. The word root-combining form for glucose is

glyc/o   _____/___.

2

Glycogen is the body's reserve food supply of glucose. To be usable glycogen must be con-

glucose   verted to _____.

3

glyc/o/gen   Glucose is usable sugar, but before it becomes
glycogen   usable it is stored in the body as
gli' ko jen   _____/____/_____.

4

Glyc/emia means sugar in the blood. Hyper/

too much sugar   glyc/emia means ** _____
  in the blood
  (high blood sugar)   _____.

hypo/glyc/emia   Write the word that means low blood sugar:
hypoglycemia
hi po gli se' mi a   _____/_____/_____.

5

The testicles are the organs in which the male
germ cells are formed; that is, spermatozoa

testicles   are formed in the _____.

6

Orchid/algia means pain in the testicle.

Orchid/ectomy means ** _____

excision of
  a testicle   _____.

7

Build a word meaning:

orchid/o/pex/y   fixation of a testicle,
orchidopexy
or' kid o peks i   _____/____/_____/___;

orchid/otomy   incision into a testicle
orchidotomy
or kid ot' o mi   _____/_____.

8
A crypt/ic remark is one with a hidden meaning. A crypt/ic belief is one whose meaning is
obscure. The word root for hidden or obscure

crypt   is _____.

9
Around the time of birth the testicles normally
descend from the abdominal cavity into the
scrotum. Sometimes this fails to happen and
the testicles are not evident. This condition is

crypt/orchid/ism
cryptorchidism   called _____/_____/ ism.
kript or' kid ism   (hidden)   (testicle)

10
When a testicle is hidden in the abdominal
cavity, the condition is known as

cryptorchidism   _____.

orchid/o/pex/y
  or   The operation to repair the condition is
orchid/o/plast/y
                        _____/____/_____/__.

11
Colp/o is used in words about the vagina.

                        Colpitis means ** _____
inflammation
  of the vagina   _____.

12
A colp/o/spasm is a ** _____

vaginal spasm   _____.

colp/otomy
colpotomy   Incision into the vagina is a
kol pot' to mi
                        _____/_____.

13

Build a word meaning:

surgical repair of the vagina,

colp/o/plast/y
(you pronounce)

_____ / / _____ / ___ ;

suture of the vagina,

colp/orrhaphy

_____ / _____ ;

instrument for examing the vagina,

colp/o/scop/e

_____ / / _____ / ___ .

The following chart is for use in building words through frame 33.

COMBINING FORM OF LOCATION	MEANING
Ect/o	Outer - outside
End/o	Inner - inside
Mes/o	Middle
Retr/o	Backward - behind
Par/a	Around - near

14

The blast/o/derm is an embryonic disk of cells that gives rise to the three main layers of tissue in man. The outer germ layer is called the ect/o/derm. The inner germ layer is called

end/o/derm
endoderm
en' do derm

the _____ / / _____ .

15

Between the ectoderm and endoderm is a middle germ layer called the

mes/o/derm
mesoderm
mes' o derm

_____ / / _____ .

16

The ectoderm forms the skin. The nervous system arises from the same layer as the skin. That is, sense organs are formed from the

ect/o/derm
ectoderm
ek' to derm

_____ / / _____ .

17
The inner germ layer forms organs inside the body. The stomach and small intestine arise

endoderm   from the _____.

18
The skeleton arises from the germ layer between the ectoderm and endoderm. Muscles,

mesoderm   too, are formed by the _____.

19
Bones and cartilages also arise from the

mesoderm   _____.

20
The blastoderm gives rise to the three germ layers. They are:

ectoderm   outer _____;

mesoderm   middle _____;

endoderm   inner _____.

21

ect/o/genous   Something produced within an organism is said
ectogenous   to be end/o/genous. Something produced out-
ek toj' in us   side an organism is _____/___/_____.

22

end/o/cyst/ic   Ect/o/cyt/ic is an adjective meaning outside a
endocystic   cell. An adjective meaning inside a bladder is
en' do sis tic   _____/___/_____/_____.

23
Prot/o/plasm is the substance of life. Ect/o/
plasm forms the outer limit of the cell. Pro-
toplasm within the cell is called

end/o/plasm   _____/___/_____.
(you pronounce)

24

End/o/crani/al is an adjective meaning within the cranium. An adjective meaning within the

end/o/cardi/al
(or referring to the
lining of the heart)

heart is _____ / / _____ / ____.

25

Build a word meaning:

examination by looking within,

end/o/scop/y

_____ / / _____ / __;

end/o/card/itis
(you pronounce)

inflammation of the lining of the heart,

_____ / / _____ / ____.

26

Ectopic means out of (the normal) place. An ectopic pregnancy occurs outside the uterus. A heart on the right side of the body is an

ectopic
ek top' ik

_____ heart.

27

If development of a fertilized embryo occurs in the abdominal cavity instead of in the uterus,

ectopic

it is called an _____ pregnancy.

28

Refer back to the chart for help. Build an adjective meaning:

behind the colon,

retr/o/col/ic
re tro kol' ik

_____ / / _____ / __;

behind the mammary (gland),

retr/o/mammary
re tro mam' ma ri

_____ / / mammary __;

behind the stern/um,

retr/o/stern/al
re tro ster' nal

_____ / / _____ / al __.

29
Ante/version means turning forward.   The word for turning backward is

retr/o/version
(you pronounce)
_____ / / _____.

30
The retr/o/periton/eum is the space

behind
_____ the peritoneum. An inflam-

retr/o/periton/itis
re tro per i to ni' tis
mation of this space is called

_____ / / _____ / _____.

31
Ant/e/flexion means forward bending. Retr/o/

backward bending
flexion means ** _____.

32
Refer to the chart again. Par/a/centr/al

near the center or
around the center
means ** _____

_____.

inflammation around
the appendix
Par/a-/appendic/itis means ** _____

_____.

33
Build a word meaning:

par/a/cyst/itis
par a sis ti' tis
inflammation around the bladder,

_____ / / _____ / _____;

par/a/colp/itis
par a kol pi' tis
inflammation of tissues around the vagina,

_____ / / _____ / _____;

par/a/nephr/itis
par a nef ri' tis
inflammation of tissues around the kidney,

_____ / / _____ / _____.

34

outer   Ect/o means _____.

inner   End/o means _____.

middle   Mes/o means _____.

around (near)   Par/a means _____.

behind   Retr/o means _____.

35
Aut/o is a word root-combining form that
means self. You already recognize auto in
such ordinary English words as aut/o/mobile
(a self-propelled vehicle) and aut/o/bi/o/

self   graph/y. Aut/o means _____.

36
Aut/o is a word root-combining form meaning
self. Aut/o/di/a/gnos/is means

diagnosing one's
own disease   ** _____.

37
Aut/o/nom/ic means self-controlling. Aut/o/

self-destruction or
self-destroying   lys/is means ** _____.

38
Mon/o means one or single. A mon/o/graph
deals with a single subject. A mon/o/nucle/ar

one   cell has _____ nucleus.

39
Mult/i means the opposite of mon/o. Mult/i

many or more
than one   means ** _____.

40
Something that is mult/i/capsular has

many capsules   * _____.

41
Par/o is the word root-combining form for
bear (give birth to). What is a mult/i/par/a

a woman who has
borne more than
one child

(pronounced mul tip' a ra)? ** _____

_____ .

42
When desiring to indicate that a woman has
born more than one child, use the noun

mult/i/par/a
multipara
mul tip' a ra

_____ / / _____ / __ .

43
Null/i means none. To nullify something is to
bring it to nothing. There are not many medical words using null/i, but when you do see it

it means _____ .

null/i/par/a
nullipara
nul ip' a ra

44
A woman who has never borne a child is a

_____ / / _____ / __ .

45
Give a meaning for each of the following:

a woman who has
never borne a child

nullipara (noun) ** _____

_____ ;

(describes) never
having borne a child

nulliparous (adjective) ** _____

_____ ;

condition of never
having borne a child

nulliparity (noun) ** _____

_____ .

46
Give a word root-combining form for:

null/i

mon/o

mult/i

par/o

none _____ / __ ;

one (single) _____ / __ ;

many _____ / __ ;

bear _____ / __ .

PREFIXES OF PLACE

These prefixes often cause difficulty in word building because of their
similarity. The explanations should be helpful. These forms will probably require extra work; this is your first introduction to prefixes of
place. Use this information carefully while working through frame 61.

PREFIX	MEANING	SENSE OF MEANING
Ab	From	Away from (absence)
De	From	Down from or from - resulting in less than (descent)
Ex	From	Out from (exit)

47
You have already learned ab as the opposite of
ad; ad means toward, ab means

from or
  away from

_____ .

48
Build a word that means

moving away from the midline,

ab/duct/ion

_____ / _____ / _____ ;

moving away from the normal,

ab/norm/al

_____ / _____ / _____ .

49

away from | Ab/errant means wandering *_____
the normal course. Ab/ort means taking the

away from | fetus *_____ the mother.

50

from or down from | The prefix de also means _____.

51

When one de/scends the stairs, he comes down
from a higher level. A de/scending nerve

down from | track comes *_____ the brain.

52

A de/coction is a boiled down, thicker substance because water has been taken

from | _____ it.

53

When water is taken from a substance, the substance is less than it was. Write a word that
means to remove the water from a substance.

dehydration
or dehydrate | _____.

de/hydr/ation
dehydration
de hi dra' shun

54

When water is taken from a cell,

_____/_____/_____ occurs.

de/hydr/ated
de hi' dra ted

55

When water is lost from the body because of
excessive vomiting, the patient is

_____/_____/_____.

decalcification
de kal si fi ka' shun

56

When calcium is removed from the bones,
there is less calcium than before. This

process is called _____/ calcification ___.

57
When a pregnant woman does not eat enough
calcium for the growing baby, her own bones
will be robbed of calcium and

decalcification   _____ will occur.

58
The prefix ex also means from, but in the

out from   sense of (hint: exit) *_____.

59
Ex/eresis means the taking out (from) any part
of the body. To excise is to remove a part or

out   cut it _____.

60
To exhale is to breathe out waste matter

from   _____ the body.

61
Ex/cretion is the process of expelling (or get-
ting out from the body) a substance. Expelling
excretion
(you pronounce)   urine is urinary _____.

62
Try to work this summary frame without
referring to the chart. Give the prefix meaning from in the following sense:

ab   away from ____

ex   out from ____

de   down from or from, resulting in less than ____

63
Narc/o is the word root-combining form for
sleep. A narc/o/tic is a drug that produces
narc/o/tic   sleep. Opium produces sleep. Opium is a
narcotic
nar kot' ic   _____/ /_____.

64
A narcotic should be used only when prescribed
by a physician. Codeine produces sleep.
Opium produces sleep. Opium is a

narcotic

_____.

narc/osis
narcosis
nar ko' sis

65
The condition induced by narcotics is called

_____/_____.

66
Narc/o/leps/y means seizure or attacks of
sleep. When a person is absolutely unable to
stay awake, he suffers from

narc/o/leps/y
narcolepsy
nar' ko lep si

_____/____/_____/___.

67
A cerebroma, cerebral arteriosclerosis, and
paresis are causes of sleep seizure, called

narcolepsy

_____.

68
Is/o is used in words to mean equal. Something that is is/o/metr/ic has dimensions that

equal

are _____.

69
Blood serum has the same osmotic pressure,
or tonicity, as the red blood cells in it. Blood

is/o/ton/ic
isotonic
i so ton' ic

serum is therefore an _____/____/ ton / ic
solution.

70
Any solution that does not destroy red blood
cells, because there is no pressure difference,

isotonic

is an _____ solution.

71

Build a word meaning:

fingers or toes of equal length,

is/o/dactyl/ism   _____ / / _____ / ism ;

is/o/therm/al (or ic)   pertaining to equal temperature,
(you pronounce)   _____ / / _____ / _____ .

Use the following information to work frames 72 through 81. This is another group of prefixes of place.

PREFIX	MEANING	DIFFERENTIATION
Di/a	Through	Use with the word root-combining forms you know; used more in medical terminology
Per	Through	Prefix from Latin; used in ordinary English
Peri	Around	Prefix from Greek used with the word root-combining forms you know; used more in medical terminology
Circum	Around	Latin prefix used in ordinary English

72

Peri/articular means around articulations or joints. Peri/tonsill/ar means

around the tonsil   ** _____ .

Peri/col/ic means ** _____

around the colon   _____ .

Peri/dent/al means ** _____

around a tooth
(teeth)   _____ .

73

Another prefix that means around is

circum   _____ .

74

around

around

Circum/ocular means _____ the eyes. Circum/or/al means _____ the mouth.

75

circumscribed

sir' kum scrib d

Circum/scribed means limited in space (as though a line were drawn around it). A hive, or skin wheal, is limited in space; it does not spread. A hive may be described as a

_____ wheal.

76

circumscribed

A boil is also limited in the space it covers.

A boil is a _____ lesion.

77

circum/duct/ion
circumduction
sir kum duk' shun

Ad/duct/ion is moving towards. Ab/duct/ion is moving away. Moving around (circular

motion) is _____/_____/_____.

78

di/a

di/a/rrhea

di/a/therm/al
      (or /ic)

There are two prefixes that mean through. The one that you would expect to use more

often in medical terminology is _____/____.
Build a word meaning:
flowing through (drop the o),

_____/___/_____;
pertaining to heating through,

_____/___/_____/_____.

79

through

through

Per/for/ation (noun) means puncturing

_____. To per/for/ate means to

puncture or make a hole _____.

80

An ulcer that has eaten through the stomach

perforated   wall has _____ (past tense)
it.

81

When ulcers eat through an organ, the result

per/for/ation   is called _____/_____/ation (noun).

82

Summarize the following:
Two prefixes meaning through are _____

per and di/a   and _____/____. Two prefixes meaning around

circum and peri   are _____ and _____.

83

Necr/o is used in words pertaining to death.

death   Necr/o/cyt/osis is cellular _____.

84

Necr/osis refers to a condition in which dead
tissue is surrounded with healthy tissue. Cer-

necr/osis
necrosis   tain diseases can cause _____/_____
nek ro' sis   of the bones.

85

When blood supply is cut off from an arm, gangrene sets in. This results in

necrosis   _____ (death) of the arm tissue.

86

When gangrene occurs anywhere in the body,

necrosis   _____ is seen.

87

abnormal
  or unusual

Phil/ia is the opposite of phob/ia. Phobia is

abnormal fear of. Philia is ** _____
attraction to.

88

abnormal attraction
  to dead bodies

Necr/o/phob/ia is an abnormal fear of dead

bodies. Necr/o/phil/ia is ** _____

_____ .

89

Words that can end in phob/ia can end in phil/
ia. Abnormal fear of water is

hydr/o/phob/ia

_____ / / _____ / _____ .
Abnormal attraction to water is

hydr/o/phil/ia

_____ / / _____ / _____ .

90

Think of the meaning while building words
opposite to:
hemat/o/phob/ia,

hemat/o/phil/ia

_____ / / _____ / _____ ;
pyr/o/phob/ia,

pyr/o/phil/ia

_____ / / _____ / _____ ;
aer/o/phob/ia,

aer/o/phil/ia

_____ / / _____ / _____ ;
aut/o/phil/ia
(you pronounce)

aut/o/phob/ia,

_____ / / _____ / _____ .

91

attraction to,
  liking, or
  loving

Phil/o is the word root-combining form that

means ** _____

_____ .

92

Hom/o in words means same. Hom/o/genized milk has the same amount of cream throughout. Hom/o/gland/ular means pertaining to the

same gland   *_____.

93

hom/o/sex/ual   When men are attracted to other men much
homosexual   more than to women, they are said to be
ho mo sex' u al   _____/ /_____/_____.

94

When women are attracted to other women
rather than to men, they too are called

homosexual   _____.

95

Heter/o is the opposite of hom/o. Heter/o

different   means **_____.

96

different   Heter/opia means _____
                          vision in each eye.

97

Heter/o/trich/osis means having hair of many

different   _____ colors.

98. Look up the meaning of homogeneous and
heterogeneous in your dictionary. Explain the
difference between them.

homogeneous: orig-   **_____
  inating from with-
  in the same body   _____.

heterogeneous: **_____
  originating from
  outside the body   _____.

99
Think of their meaning while you form opposites
of the following:
hom/o/lys/is,

heter/o/lys/is

_____/   /_____/_____;

hom/o/genesis,

heter/o/genesis

_____/   /_____;

hom/o/sex/ual,

heter/o/sex/ual

_____/   /_____/_____.

100
Splen/o is used in words about the spleen.
Build a word meaning:
excision of the spleen,

splen/ectomy
sple nek' to mi

_____/_____;

enlargement of the spleen,

splen/o/megal/y

_____/   /_____/___;

hemorrhage from the spleen,

splen/orrhagia

_____/   •_____.

101
Write a meaning for:
splen/algia,

pain in the spleen

**_____;

splen/o/megaly,

enlargement
 of the spleen

**_____;

splen/ic,

pertaining to
 the spleen

**_____.

102
Syn and sym are different forms of the same

together or
 joined

prefix; syn and sym mean _____.

103

The prefix sym is the form to be used when it is followed by the consonants b, m, or p; syn is used in all other cases. Write the prefix for each of the following:

synarthrosis	_____ arthrosis,
symmetrical	_____ metrical,
symbolism	_____ bolism,
symphysis	_____ physis,
syndrome	_____ drome,
sympathy	_____ pathy.
symbiosis	_____ biosis

together

104

Both syn and sym mean _____;
sym is used when followed by the letters

b, m, p

___, ___, and ___; syn is used in other medical words.

105

Super means beyond. What does supernumerary mean? **_____

beyond the
  usual number

_____.

106

Supra means above. What does suprapubic

above the pubis

mean? **_____.
What does suprarenal mean?

above the kidney

**_____.

107

The prefixes a and an mean without.   Examine the following words:

an/al/ges/ia	a/bi/o/tic
an/aph/ia	a/blast/em/ic
an/em/ia	a/clamp/sia
an/encephal/us	a/derm/ia
an/esthes/ia	a/febrile
an/iso/cyt/osis	a/galact/ia
an/idr/osis	a/kinesi/a
an/irid/ia	a/lali/a
an/onych/ia	a/men/ia
an/op/ia	a/pne/a
an/ur/ia	a/reflex/ia
an/ur/esis	a/seps/is

Draw a conclusion.   When the prefix is followed

a   by a consonant, use _____ .
                              (a, an)
When the prefix is followed by a vowel, use

an   _____ .
         (a, an)

In this unit you worked with more than 60 new medical terms.
Fifty of them are listed here for you to practice your pronunciation.
Do that now.   Then take the Unit 7 Self-Test.

abduction	endoplasm	orchidopexy
abort	endoscopy	para-appendicitis
aerophobia	excretion	paracolpitis
autodiagnosis	glycogen	paracystitis
autophobia	hematophobia	peridental
circumduction	heterogeneous	peritonsillar
circumocular	heterosexual	pyrophobia
colporrhaphy	homosexual	retrocolic
colpospasm	isocellular	retroperitonitis
colpotomy	isotonic	retrosternal
cryptorchidism	mesoderm	retroversion
decalcification	mononuclear	splenomegaly
dehydration	multipara	symbiosis
ectoderm	narcolepsy	synergetic
ectogenous	necrophobia	supernumerary
ectopic	nulliparity	suprarenal
endocarditis	orchidalgia	

UNIT 7   SELF-TEST

From the list on the right select the correct meaning for each of the following often-used medical terms:

_____	1. Paracolpitis	a.	Condition of undescended testicle
_____	2. Narcolepsy	b.	A location behind the sternum
_____	3. Dehydration	c.	Abnormal fear of death
_____	4. Heterosexual	d.	Beyond the usual number
_____	5. Abort	e.	An uncontrollable condition of falling asleep
_____	6. Cryptorchidism		
_____	7. Multipara	f.	Spasm of the vagina
_____	8. Isotonic	g.	A condition of living together
_____	9. Colpospasm	h.	Abnormal fear of being alone
_____	10. Autophobia	i.	Out of the usual location
_____	11. Supernumerary	j.	Having the same osmotic pressure
_____	12. Retrosternal	k.	Relating to around the tonsil
_____	13. Peritonsillar	l.	One who is attracted to people of the same sex
_____	14. Ectopic		
_____	15. Mononuclear	m.	A condition of having had water removed from

n. Inflammation around the bladder

o. Having one nucleus

p. One who is attracted to people of the other sex

q. Inflammation around the vagina

r. A woman who has borne more than one child

s. Taking the fetus away from the mother's womb

PART 2

Complete each of the medical terms on the right with the missing part(s):

1.	Relating to around the eye	_____ocular
2.	Movement away from the midline	_____ duction
3.	Pertaining to being out of the normal place	_____
4.	One who is attracted to people of the same sex	_____
5.	The form in which glucose is stored in the body	_____ gen
6.	The outermost layer of skin	_____ derm
7.	Surgical fixation of the testicle	_____ pexy
8.	Abnormally enlarged spleen	_____
9.	Abnormal fear of blood	Hemato _____
10.	The condition of never having borne a child	_____parity
11.	Diagnosing one's own illness	_____
12.	Pertaining to around the teeth	_____
13.	Inflammation behind the peritoneal cavity	_____ periton _____
14.	Suturing of the vagina	_____
15.	Relating to working together	_____ erget _____

ANSWERS

Part 1

1.	q	9.	f
2.	e	10.	h
3.	m	11.	d
4.	p	12.	b
5.	s	13.	k
6.	a	14.	i
7.	r	15.	o
8.	j		

Part 2

1. Circumocular
2. Abduction
3. Ectopic
4. Homosexual
5. Glycogen
6. Ectoderm
7. Orchidopexy
8. Splenomegaly
9. Hematophobia
10. Nulliparity
11. Autodiagnosis
12. Peridental
13. Retroperitonitis
14. Colporrhaphy
15. Synergetic

Unit 8

In this unit you will add new prefixes to many combining forms you have already used. Altogether you will put together more than 100 new medical terms. The new word parts you will use are <u>metr/o</u> (uterus), <u>sanguin/o</u> (blood relationship), and the following:

<u>ante</u> (before, forward)	<u>infra</u> (under, below)
<u>anti</u> (against)	<u>intra</u> (within)
<u>bi</u> (two)	<u>mal</u> (bad, poor)
<u>con</u> (with)	<u>post</u> (behind, after)
<u>contra</u> (against)	<u>pre</u> (before, in front of)
<u>dis</u> (free of)	<u>semi</u> (half, partial)
<u>epi</u> (upon, over)	<u>sub</u> (under)
<u>extra</u> (outside of)	<u>trans</u> (across)
<u>hemi</u> (half)	<u>tri</u> (three)
<u>in</u> (in, not)	<u>uni</u> (one)

You will also have some practice in making plural words from the singular form and forming the singular of some plural forms.

1

Hyster/o is used in words about the uterus. Metr/o is another word root-combining form

uterus   that refers to the _____.

2

Hyster/o usually refers to the uterus as an organ. Metr/o usually refers to the tissues

uterus   of the _____.

3

There are exceptions to the rule, but in general hyster/o means the uterus as an

organ   _____. Metr/o refers to the uterus

tissues   in the sense of its _____.

4

Metr/itis means an inflammation of the uterine musculature. Metr/o/paralysis means paraly-

uterus or   sis of the ** _____
  uterine musculature   _____.

5

Using metr/orrhagia as an example, build a word meaning:

metr/orrhea   flow or discharge from the uterus,
met ror re' a   _____/_____;

metr/orrhexis   rupture of the uterus,
met ro reks' is   _____/_____;

metr/o/path/y   any uterine disease,
  or hysteropathy   _____/__/_____/___;

metr/o/cele   herniation of the uterus,
  or hysterocele   _____/__/_____.

6

The end/o/metr/ium is the lining of the uterus or, literally, the inner tissues of the uterus. Build a word meaning:

end/o/metr/itis   inflammation of the uterine lining,
en do me tri' tis   _____/__/_____/_____;

end/o/metr/ectomy   excision of the uterine lining,
en do me trek' to me   _____/__/_____/_____.

More prefixes! Use this chart to work frames 7 through 20.

PREFIX	MEANING	SPECIAL COMMENT
Epi	Over – upon	
Extra	Outside Beyond In addition to	
Infra	Below – under	Almost always below a part of the body Almost always adjectival in form There are fewer words beginning with infra than with sub
Sub	Under – below	Many words of all kinds begin with sub

7
The epi/gastr/ic region is the region

over the stomach   ** _____.

8
Epi/splen/itis means inflammation of the

over the spleen   tissue ** _____.

9
Build a word meaning:

excision of the tissue on the kidney,

epi/nephr/ectomy
ep i ne frek' to mi   _____ / _____ / _____ ;

suture of the region over the stomach,

epi/gastr/orrhaphy
ep i gas tror' a fi   _____ / _____ / _____ .

10
Use the chart if you need help. Extra/nuclear

outside or beyond   means ** _____ a nucleus.

11

outside or beyond   Extra/uterine means ** _____
the uterus.

12
Give a meaning for each of the following:

outside or beyond   extragenital ** _____
the genitals   _____;

outside or beyond   extrahepatic ** _____
the liver   _____;

outside or beyond the   extramarginal ** _____
edges or margins   _____.

13
Refer to the chart; infra is a prefix that means

below or under   _____.

14
below or under   Infra/mammary means _____
the mammary gland.

15
below or under   Infra/patell/ar means _____
the patella (knee-cap).

16
below or under   The prefix sub also means _____.

17
under   Sub/abdominal means _____ the abdo-

below   men. Sub/aur/al means _____ the ear.

18

The prefixes infra and sub are sometimes con-
fusing in word building. For that reason you
will build words that can take either prefix.
When you see sub or infra, you will think of

below or under   _____ or _____ .

19

Using stern/o, build two words meaning below
the sternum (breast bone):

infra/stern/al   _____/_____/_____ ;

sub/stern/al   _____/_____/_____ .

A word meaning above the sternum is

supra/stern/al   __supra__/_____/_____ .

20

Using pub/o, build two words meaning under
the pubis:

infra/pub/ic   _____/_____/_____ ;

sub/pub/ic   _____/_____/_____ .

A word meaning above the pubis is

supra/pub/ic   _____/_____/_____ .

21

The prefix anti means against. An anti/pyretic

against   is an agent that works _____ a
fever. An anti/narcotic is an agent that works

against   _____ narcotics.

22
Build an adjective describing an agent that
works against:

rheumatic disease,

anti/rheumatic   _____/_____;

spastic disease,

anti/spastic   _____/_____;

anti/syphilitic   syphilitic infections,
(you pronounce)   _____/_____.

23
Build an adjective describing an agent that
works against:

convulsive states,

anti/convulsive   _____/_____;

arthritic diseases,

anti/arthritic   _____/_____;

anti/toxic   toxic states,
(you pronounce)   _____/_____.

24
The prefix contra also means against; contra is
used with modern English words. To contra/

against   dict someone is to speak _____
                       what he is saying.

25
against   Contra/ry things are _____ one
                       another. A contra/ry person is usually one who

against   is _____ your wishes.

26

In medical terminology contra is mainly con-
fined in use to only four words.   Give a meaning for each of the following:

contraindication,

indication
against

** _____;

against
conceiving

contraceptive,

** _____;

against
one's will

contravolitional,

** _____;

against the side
(you pronounce)

contralateral,

** _____.

27

Form a word for each of the following:

contravolitional

against one's will, _____;

contraindication

against indication, _____;

contraceptive

against conception, _____;

contralateral
(you pronounce)

against the side, _____.

28

Using the noun given, build the other parts of
the same word:

| contra | / | indicat | / | ion | (noun); |

contra/indicat/e

_____ / _____ / _____ (verb);

contra/indicat/ed
(you pronounce)

_____ / _____ / _____ (past
tense).

29

The prefix trans means across or over.   To

across or over

trans/port a cargo is to carry it _____
the ocean or land.

30
Trans/position means literally position

across or over   _____ .

31
Transposition means literally placed across.
When an organ is placed across to the other
trans/position   side of the body (whence it is normally found)
transposition
trans po zi' shun   _____/_____ occurs.

32
Cardi/ac transposition means that the heart is
on the right side of the body. If the stomach is
on the right side of the body, the condition is
transposition   gastr/ic _____ .

33
When a trans/fusion is given, blood is passed

across or over   _____ from one person to another.

34
The prefix in means in or not. Incompatible

not   drugs are drugs that do _____ mix with each
other. In/compet/ency occurs in an organ when

not   it is _____ able to perform its function.

35
When the ile/o/cec/al valve cannot perform its
in/compet/ency   function, the result is ileocecal
incompetency
in com' pe ten si   _____/_____/_____ .

36
When a person is not able to take care of him-
self, you refer to it as ment/al

incompetency   _____ . You may even

incompetent   say the person is mentally _____ .
                                        (adjective)

37
Write a meaning for each of the following:

not sane | insane ** _____ ;

unable to sleep | insomnia ** _____ ;

not sanitary (clean) | insanitary ** _____ .

in/cis/ion
incision
in sizh' un

38
The prefix in means not but it also means in.
To in/cis/e is to cut into. This is a verb. The

noun from in/cis/e is _____ / _____ / _____ .

39
Breathing is respiration. Breathing consists of
the following two processes. Define them:

breathing out or the
act of carrying
water vapors and
waste gases to the
outside of the body

expiration ** _____

_____

_____ ;

breathing in or the
act of taking in
essential gases

inspiration ** _____

_____ .

40
The prefix in may have either of two meanings.

not or in | It may mean _____ or _____ .

41
Mal is a French word that means bad; mal is
also a prefix that means bad or poor. Mal/

bad | odor/ous means having a _____ odor.

42
Mal/aise means a general feeling of illness or
poor feeling. Mal/form/ation means

poorly formed or
poor formation

** _____ .

43
Mal/nutrition means ** _____

poor nutrition _____.

bad (abnormal) posi-
tion or placement

Mal/position means ** _____

_____.

Below is a chart that shows some of the prefixes of quantity. Use it
while working frames 44 through 52.

PREFIX	MEANING	EXPLANATION
Uni	One	
Bi	Two Double	
Tri	Three	
Semi	Half	Used with modern English words or words closer to modern English
Hemi	Half	Used more with straight medical words

44

three   The tri/ceps muscle has _____ heads.

two   A bi/cusp/id is a tooth with _____ cusps.

one   A uni/corn has _____ horn.

45
Later/al means pertaining to the side. Build a
word meaning pertaining to:

uni/later/al   one side, _____/_____/_____;

bi/later/al   two sides, _____/_____/_____;

tri/later/al   three sides, _____/_____/____.
(you pronounce)

46
A tri/later/al figure looks like △ .

tri/angle

You call this a _____/_____.

47
What word would you use to describe something made of only one cell

uni/cell/ular
(you pronounce)

_____/_____/_____,

but having two nucle/i ?

bi/nucle/ar
(you pronounce)

_____/_____/_____.

48
To bi/furc/ate is to divide into two forks.
When an artery divides into two, it

bi/furc/ates
bifurcates
bi' fur kates

_____/_____/_____ (s).

49
Bifurcate is a verb.   The noun is bifurcation.
When a nerve divides into two branches, a

bifurcation
bi fur ka' shun

_____ (noun) is formed.

50

one

uni means _____;

two

bi means _____;

three

tri means _____;

many

mult/i means _____.

51
There are two prefixes that mean half: semi and hemi. Using semi, form a word that means:

semi/circle

half circle, _____/_____;

semi/conscious

half conscious, _____/_____;

semi/private
(you pronounce)

half private, _____/_____.

52

Using hemi, build a word meaning:

having only half a heart (noun),

hemi/cardi/a

_____/_____/____ ;

hemi/pleg/ia
(hemi/paralysis)
(you pronounce)

paralysis of half the body,

_____/_____/ ia   .

53

The prefix con means with. A.child who has

with

con/genit/al cataracts was born _____
cataracts.

54

con/genit/al
congenital
con jen' i tal

A child born with a lateral curvature of the
spine has a deformity called

_____/_____/_____ scoliosis.

55

Another way of saying born with a deformity is
to say congenital anomaly. A child born hump-

congenital

backed has a _____ anomaly.

56

congenital

A child born with syphilis has _____
syphilis.

57

con/sanguin/ity
consanguinity
kon san gwin' it i

con – prefix, with;
sanguin/o – combining form, blood;
ity – noun suffix.
Using what you need of these word parts, build
a word meaning literally with blood or in usage,
blood relationship:

_____/_____/_____ .

58

Con/sanguin/ity is a relationship by descent from a common ancestor. The noun that expresses the relationship of cousins is

consanguinity   _____.

sanguin/al
sanguinal
sang' gwin al

59

Sanguin/o means bloody. Build a word meaning

pertaining to blood: _____ / ____.

60

The prefix dis means to free of or to undo.

Dis/ease means literally ** _____

to free of ease   _____.

61

To dis/sect is to cut a tissue or to undo it (into parts) for purposes of study. Write a meaning for each of the following:

to make free
  from infection

disinfect ** _____

_____;

to undo from
  association

disassociate ** _____

_____.

62

to free of,
  to undo

The prefix dis means ** _____

_____.

with

The prefix con means _____.

Use the following chart to work frames 63 through 68.

PREFIX	MEANING	SPECIFIC COMMENTS
Post	Behind After	
Ante	Before Forward	Few usages
Pre	Before In front of	Many usages

63
Refer to the chart. Post/cibal means

after   _____ meals. Post/esophageal means

behind   _____ the esophagus.

64

before   Try it again. Pre/an/esthetic means _____
                anesthesia. Pre/hyoid means

in front of   *_____ the hyoid bone.

65

before   Once again. Ante/pyretic means _____

in front of   the fever. Pre/hyoid means *_____
                the hyoid bone.

66
Nat/al means birth. Give a meaning for each
of the following:

after birth   postnatal *_____;

before birth   prenatal *_____;

before birth   antenatal *_____.

67
Febr/ile means fever.   Write a meaning for:

after a fever   postfebrile *_____;

before a fever   antefebrile *_____.

68
Give the meaning of each of the following:

after surgery   postoperative *_____;

behind the uterus   postuterine *_____;

before surgery   preoperative *_____;

in front of the frontal   prefrontal *_____
  lobe of the brain
                       _____;

turning forward   anteversion *_____;

before meals   antecibal *_____.

69
within the   Intr/a means within.   Intr/a-/abdominal means
  abdomen
                       *_____.

70
Build an adjective meaning:

intra-arterial   within an artery _____;

intracranial   within the cranium _____;

intravenous   within a vein _____.

The following chart contains information about the formation of plurals from the singular.   Use it to work frames 71 through 81.

TO FORM PLURALS

If the singular ending is	The plural ending is
a	ae (pronounce ae as i)
us	i
um	a
ma	mata
on	a
is	es
ix	ices ⎫ The word root is usually built
ex	ices ⎬ from the plural forms of words
ax	aces ⎭ ending in ix, ex, and ax (e.g., radix, radic/es radic/otomy radic/i/form).

71

Form the plural of:

bursae
bur' si

bursa _____;

conjuctivae
con junk ti' vi

conjunctiva _____;

bacilli
ba sil' i

bacillus _____.

72

Give the singular of:

vertebra
ver te bra

vertebrae _____;

nucleus
noo' kli us

nuclei _____;

cornea
kor' nea

corneae _____.

73
Form the plural of:

atria
a' tria   atrium _____;

cocci
kok' si   coccus _____;

ilea
(you pronounce)   ileum _____.

74
Give the singular of:

enema
en' e ma   enemata _____;

bacterium   bacteria _____;

ovum   ova _____.
(you pronounce)

75
Form the plural of:

cortices
kor' ti ses   cortex _____;

fibromata
fi bro' ma ta   fibroma _____;

protozoa
pro to zo' a   protozoon _____.

76
Give the singular of:

stigma
stig' ma   stigmata _____;

prognosis
prog' no' sis   prognoses _____;

spermatozoon
sper mat' o zo on   spermatozoa _____.

77

Form the plural of:

appendices
(you pronounce)

appendix _____ ;

diagnoses
di ag no' ses

diagnosis _____ ;

ganglia
gang' li a

ganglion _____ .

78

Refer to the chart. Give the word root that
usually refers to:

appendic

the appendix _____ ;

cortic

the cortex _____ ;

thorac
(you pronounce)

the thorax _____ .

79

The combining form of the word roots you just
discovered takes the o. These word roots
become:

appendic/o

appendic _____ / ____ ;

cortic/o

cortic _____ / ____ ;

thorac/o

thorac _____ / ____ .

80

With this new knowledge, which you found for
yourself, build a word meaning:

appendic/itis
ap pen di si' tis

inflammation of the appendix,

_____ / _____ ;

cortic/al
kor' tic al

pertaining to the cortex,

_____ / _____ ;

thorac/o/centesis
tho rak o sen te' sis

surgical puncture of the thorax,

_____ / ____ / _____ .

81
Form the plural of:

apices   apex _____ ;

fornices   fornex _____ ;

varices   varix _____ ;

sarcomata   sarcoma _____ ;

septa   septum _____ ;

radii   radius _____ ;

maxillae   maxilla _____ .
(you pronounce)

82
There are other ways of forming plurals. They
apply to only a few words. When you meet
these words and have a question about how their
plural forms are built, consult a medical dictionary.

Here are 50 of the medical terms you worked with in this unit. Pronounce each carefully, then complete Unit 8 Self-Test.

antecibal	dissect	postcibal
anteflexion	epigastric	postfebrile
antenatal	expiration	semicircular
anteversion	extrahepatic	semiconscious
antiarthritic	extrauterine	subaural
anticonvulsive	hemiplegia	substernal
antipyretic	incompetency	suprapubic
antitoxin	inframammary	suprasternal
bicuspid	infrasternal	transfusion
bilateral	insomnia	transposition
congenital	inspiration	triceps
consanguinity	intracranial	trilateral
contraceptive	intravenous	unicellular
contraindication	malnutrition	unilateral
contralateral	malposition	varix (varices)
disassociate	prenatal	vertebra
disinfect	preoperative	(vertebrae)

UNIT 8 SELF-TEST

PART 1

From the list on the right select the correct meaning for each of the following often-used medical terms:

_____ 1. Transposition

_____ 2. Unicellular

_____ 3. Semiconscious

_____ 4. Contraindication

_____ 5. Anteflexion

_____ 6. Hemiplegia

_____ 7. Extrauterine

_____ 8. Antitoxin

_____ 9. Prenatal

_____ 10. Subaural

_____ 11. Triceps

_____ 12. Postcibal

_____ 13. Malposition

_____ 14. Intracranial

_____ 15. Disassociate

a. Evidence that indicates against

b. A chemical agent that works against a toxin

c. Outside of the uterus

d. Placed across (to the other side)

e. Above the pubis

f. After having eaten

g. Relating to having a single cell

h. Bad or poor position

i. Within the cranium

j. Half or partially conscious

k. Free from association

l. Coming before the operation

m. Bending forward

n. Under the ear

o. A three-headed muscle of the upper arm

p. Before birth

q. Pertaining to over (upon) the stomach

r. Paralysis of half the body

PART 2

Complete each of the medical terms on the right with the missing part(s):

1. Inability to sleep   _____ somn _____

2. Relating to two sides   _____

3. Half or part of a circle   _____

4. Pertaining to under the breast
    bone   _____ stern _____

5. Relating to before the operation   _____

6. Having the property of acting
    against a fever   _____ pyret _____

7. Passing blood across from one
    person to another   _____

8. Relating to only one side   _____

9. A condition of poor nutrition   _____

10. Within a vein   _____venous

11. Under or below the mammary gland   _____mammary

12. A chemical agent that works against
    fertilization of the ovum   _____ive

13. A condition of not being competent   _____

14. Outside of the liver   _____hepatic

15. The condition that a person is born
    with   _____genital

ANSWERS

Part 1

1.	d	9.	p
2.	g	10.	n
3.	j	11.	o
4.	a	12.	f
5.	m	13.	h
6.	r	14.	i
7.	c	15.	k
8.	b		

Part 2

1. Insomnia
2. Bilateral
3. Semicircle
4. Substernal
5. Preoperative
6. Antipyretic
7. Transfusion
8. Unilateral

9. Malnutrition
10. Intravenous
11. Inframammary
12. Contraceptive
13. Incompetency
14. Extrahepatic
15. Congenital

Unit 9

You will put together more than 100 new medical terms in this unit. You will use what you have already covered plus the following:

acromi/o (acromion)
ankyl/o (stiffness)
bronch/i, bronch/o (bronchus)
calcane/o (calcaneous)
carp/o (carpal, wrist)
condyl/o (condyle)
dextr/o (right)
gangli/o (ganglion)
humer/o (humerus)
ischi/o (ischium)
laryng/o (larynx)
ment/o (chin)

neo- (new)

nas/o (nose)
noct/i (night)
phag/o (eat)
phalang/o (phalanges)
pharyng/o (pharynx)
pleur/o (pleura)
sinistr/o (left)
stern/o (sternum, breastbone)
thromb/o (thrombus)
trache/o (trachea)
vas/o (vessel)

-manual (hand)
-pedal (foot)
-plasm (growth)

1
Use the following information to work frames 1 through 13. If you have forgotten a word part, remember you may look back. If you don't know the anatomy of the respiratory system, look at the diagram provided for you. Seeing the parts as you work will make your work more interesting.

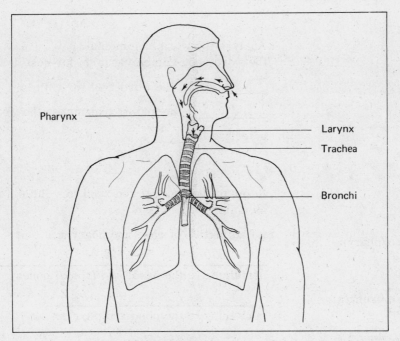

Air enters the
  nose - nas/o (Remember rhin/o ? Nas/o is
    another word meaning nose. Use it in this
    work.)
goes to the
  pharynx - pharyng/o
to the
  larynx - laryng/o
through the
  trachea - trache/o
and through the
  bronch/i (us) - bronch/o
to the
  part of the lung where it enters the
  bloodstream.
The lungs are covered by a very tough, thin
  film called the
  pleura - pleur/o.

2
Nas/o/ment/al means pertaining to the chin and

nose   _____. Write a word that means pertain-

nasal   ing to the nose. _____.

3
Analyze the word nasomental:
the word root-combining form for nose is

nas/o

_____ / ___ ; the word root for chin is

ment

_____ ; the ending that makes the word an

al

adjective is _____.

4
Refer to the chart if you need to. Build a word
meaning:

nas/o/pharyng/
   itis

inflammation of nose and pharynx,

_____ / / _____ / _____ ;

nas/o/front/al

pertaining to the nasal and frontal bones,

_____ / / _____ / ____ ;

nas/o/pharyng/eal
(you pronounce)

pertaining to the nose and pharynx,

_____ / / _____ / _____ .

5
Build a word meaning:

pharyng/itis
far in ji' tis

inflammation of the pharynx,

_____ / _____ ;

pharyng/o/plast/y
far in' go plas ti

surgical repair of the pharynx,

_____ / / _____ / ___ ;

pharyng/otomy
far in got' o mi

incision of the pharynx,

_____ / _____ .

6
Look again at the chart. A laryng/o/cele is a

herniation of
   the larynx

** _____ .

7
Build a word meaning:

pertaining to the larynx,

laryngeal
_____;

instrument used to examine the larynx,

laryngoscope
_____;

spasm of the larynx,

laryngospasm
(you pronounce)
_____.

8
The chart may help you with this one.
Trache/orrhagia means

hemorrhage from
the trachea
** _____.

9
Build a word meaning:

pain in the trachea,

trache/algia
tra ke al' ji a
_____/_____;

incision into the trachea,

trache/otomy
tra ke ot' o mi
_____/_____;

trach/e/al
tra' ke al
pertaining to the trachea,

_____/____/_____;

trache/o/laryng/
otomy
tra ke o la rin
got' o mi
incision of trachea and larynx,

_____/____/_____/_____.

10
Refer back to the chart.   Bronchitis means

inflammation of
the bronchi
** _____.

an instrument to
examine the
bronchi
A bronchoscope is ** _____

_____.

11

Build a word meaning:

examination of a bronchus (with instrument),

bronch/o/scop/y
bron kos' ki pi

_____ / / _____ / __ ;

bronch/orrhagia
bron kor a' ji a

bronchial hemorrhage,

_____ / _____ ;

bronch/o/spasm
(you pronounce)

spasm of a bronchus,

_____ / / _____ .

12

Pleur/al means ** _____

pertaining to the
pleura or the cov-
ering of the lungs

_____

_____ .

inflammation of
the pleura

Pleur/itis means

** _____ .

13

Build a word meaning:

pleur/algia
plu ral' ji a

pain in the pleura, _____ / _____ ;

surgical puncturing of the pleura,

pleur/o/centesis
plu ro sen te' sis

_____ / / _____ ;

pertaining to the pleura and viscer/a,

pleurovisceral

_____ ;

pleurectomy
(you pronounce)

excision of part of the pleura,

_____ .

14

The word sinister means wicked or evil. The
Latin word sinister means left or left-handed.
In medieval times, when superstition was ram-
pant, the majority of the people (who were right-
handed) considered left-handed people cursed by
the devil. Hence these unfortunate few people
became the personification of evil. This is how
sinister found its common, contemporary meaning.

15

In medicine you go back to the original meaning
of sinister to find the word root-combining

left   form, sinistr/o, which means _____.

16

                                Give the meaning for each of the following:
pertaining
  to the left   sinistr/al, ** _____;

displacement of   sinistr/o/cardi/a,
  the heart to
  the left   ** _____;

pertaining to the
  left half of the   sinistr/o/cerebr/al, ** _____
  cerebrum
                                _____.

17

                                Using manual (hand) and pedal (foot), build a
                                word meaning:
sinistromanual
                                left-handed, _____;
sinistropedal
(you pronounce)   left-footed, _____.

18

                                The opposite of sinistr/o is dextr/o. Dextr/o

right   means _____.

19

                                Build a word meaning:
dextr/al
dex' tral   pertaining to the right, _____/_____;

dextr/o/cardi/a   displacement of the heart to the right,
deks tro kar' di a
                                _____/_/_____/___;

dextr/o/gastr/ia   displacement of the stomach to the right,
deks tro gas' tri a
                                _____/_/_____/____.

20

Refer to frame 17 if necessary and build a word meaning:

dextromanual

right-handed, _____ ;

dextropedal
(you pronounce)

right-footed, _____ .

21

Vas is a word meaning vessel. Vas/o is another word root-combining form for vessel. Vas/o/dilatation means enlarging the diameter of a

vessel

_____ .

22

decreasing the size
  of the diameter of
  a vessel

The opposite of vas/o/dilatation is vas/o/con-striction, which means ** _____

_____ .

23

vas/al
va' sal

vas/o/spasm
vas' o spazm

vas/o/tripsy
vas' o trip si

Using vas/o, build a word meaning:

pertaining to a vessel, _____ / _____ ;

spasm of a vessel,

_____ / / _____ ;

crushing (trips/y) of a vessel,

_____ / / _____ .

24

vas/otomy
vas ot' o mi

vas/orrhaphy
vas or' a fi

Vas also refers to vas deferens (a vessel that carries spermatozoa from the testes to the urethra). Build a word meaning:

incision into the vas deferens,

_____ / _____ ;

suture of the vas deferens,

_____ / _____ ;

excision of a section of the vas deferens
(sterilization procedure),

vas/ectomy
vaz ec' to mi

_____ / _____ .

25
Ne/o in words means new. Ne/o/genesis means

new   regeneration of _____ tissue.

26
new   Ne/o/nat/al refers to the _____ born. A

new   ne/o/plasm is any kind of a tumor or _____
                           growth (plasm/o refers to growth).

27
ne/o/plasm   A nonmalignant tumor is called a
neoplasm
ne' o plazm   _____ / _____ / _____ . Carcinoma is a

neoplasm   _____ .

28
Build a word meaning:

ne/o/cyt/e   new cell, _____ / _____ / _____ / e ;
                           abnormal fear of new things,

ne/o/phob/ia   _____ / _____ / _____ / ___ ;

ne/o/plasm   benign tumor,
(you pronounce)
                           _____ / _____ / _____ .

29
Noct/i is the combining form that means night.
Noct/i/luca are microscopic marine animals
that make the ocean glow during the

night   _____ .

30
Those of you who have studied music know that
a noct/urne is a dreamy music, sometimes

night   called _____ music.

31
If ambulism means walking, what do you think

sleep walking or,
   literally, walk-
   ing at night

noct/ambulism means ? **_____

_____.

32
A person is not really asleep when he sleep-
walks. People appear to be asleep but are
really suppressing the memory of what they do.

noctambulism

They are indulging in _____.

33
Build words that mean:

abnormal fear of night,

noct/i/phob/ia

_____/ /_____/_____;

excessive urination during the night,

noct/i/ur/ia

_____/ /_____/_____;

noct/i/phil/ia
(you pronounce)

unusual attraction to the night,

_____/ /_____/_____.

34
Ankly/o means stiff or not movable. Ankylosed
means stiffened. Ankylosis is a condition of

stiffness

**_____.

Review the following chart and use it to build words in frame 35.

COMBINING FORM	WITH NOUN ENDING
aden/o (gland)	aden/ia
cardi/o (heart)	cardi/a
cheil/o (lips)	cheil/ia
dactyl/o (fingers)	dactyl/ia
dent/o (teeth)	dent/ia
derm/o (skin)	derm/a (ia)
gastr/o (stomach)	gastr/ia
gloss/o (tongue)	gloss/ia
ophthalm/o (eye)	ophthalm/ia
ot/o (ear)	ot/ia
pneumon/o (lung)	pneumon/ia
proct/o (anus and rectum)	proct/ia
urethr/o (urethra)	urethr/a

35
Ankyl/o/stom/a means lockjaw (stiff jaw).
Build a word meaning (remember, you may
look back):

adhesions of lips (immovable lips),

ankyl/o/cheil/ia   _____ / / _____ / ____ ;

closure (immobility) of the anus,

ankyl/o/proct/ia   _____ / / _____ / ____ ;

abnormal fear of stiffness,

ankyl/o/phob/ia   _____ / / _____ / ____ ;
(you pronounce)

tongue tied (stiff tongue),

ankyl/o/gloss/ia   _____ / / _____ / ____ .

36
Stasis is a word meaning stopping or controlling.   To say that you control an organ or control what that organ produces, use the combining form for the organ (or product) and add the

stasis   word _____ .
(you pronounce)

controls or stops	**37** A fung/i/stasis is an agent that _____ fungus growth. Lymph/o/stasis means
control	_____ of lymph flow.

38

control or stopping of bile secretion	Chol/e/stasis means ** _____ _____.
referring to the control of the growth of bacteria	Bacteri/o/statis means ** _____ _____.

39

Build a word meaning:

hem/o/stasis he mos' ta sis	controlling the flow of blood: _____ / _____ / _____ ;
phleb/o/stasis or ven/o/stasis fleb os' ta sis	checking flow in the veins, _____ / _____ / _____ ;
arter/o/stasis ar te ri os' ta sis	checking flow in the arteries, _____ / _____ / _____ .

Use the labels on the following drawing plus your dictionary to work
frames 40 through 68.

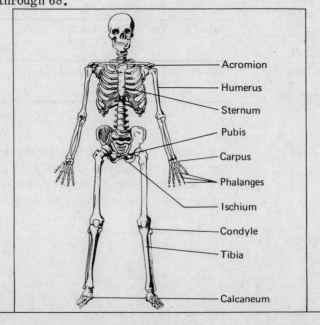

- Acromion
- Humerus
- Sternum
- Pubis
- Carpus
- Phalanges
- Ischium
- Condyle
- Tibia
- Calcaneum

foot	**40** Locate the calcaneum. This bone is found in the heel of the _____.
calcane calcane/o	**41** From calcaneum and calcanea (plural) derive the word root for the heel: _____. Give the combining form: _____.
calcane/al calcaneal kal ka' neal infra/calcane/al	**42** Now build a word meaning: pertaining to the heel, _____/_____; pertaining to below the calcaneum (infra means below or under), _____/_____/_____.
heel	**43** Calcane/o in a word refers to the _____.
carpi	**44** Locate the carpus. The plural of carpus is _____.
carp carp/o	**45** From carpus and carpi derive a word root that refers to the wrist. It is _____. The combining form is _____/___.
carp/al kar' pal carp/ectomy kar pek' to mi	**46** Build a word meaning: pertaining to the wrist (adjective), _____/_____; excision of all or part of the wrist, _____/_____.

47

wrist

Carp/o in a word refers to the _____.

Congratulations! You are now finding your own word root-combining forms. Feels good, doesn't it? Let's do some more.

48

Locate the ischium. It is part of the bony struc-

hips or pelvic
  girdle

ture that forms the ** _____

_____. The plural of ischium is

ischia

_____.

49

From ischium and ischia, derive a word root that refers to the part of the hip bone on which the body rests when sitting. The word root is

ischi

_____. The combining form that is used in words to refer to the ischium is

ischi/o

_____/___.

50

Form a word meaning:

ischi/o/rect/al
is ki o rek' tal

pertaining to the ischium and rectum,

_____/____/_____/____;

ischi/o/neur/algia
is ki o nu ral' ji a
  (or sciatica)

neuralgic pain in the hip,

_____/____/_____/_____;

ischi/o/pub/ic
is ki o pu' bic

pertaining to the ischium and pubis,

_____/____/_____/____;

ischi/al
is' ki al

pertaining to the ischium,

_____/____.

51

ischium
is' ki um

Ischi/o in a word refers to the part of the hip

bone known as the _____.

52

Locate the pubis. It is the anterior segment of

pelvic girdle

the _____.

53

pub/o (used most
  often) or pubi/o

The word root-combining form used in words

about the pubis is _____/___ .

54

pub/ic
pu' bik

Using pub/o, build a word meaning:

pertaining to the pubis, _____/_____ ;

pub/o/femor/al
pu bo fem' or al

pertaining to the pubis and femur,

_____/___/_____/___ .

55

pubis

Pub/o in a word refers to the _____ .

56

breastbone

Locate the sternum. It is often called

_____. The word root-

stern/o

combining form for sternum is _____/___ .

57

Now write a word meaning:

pertaining to the sternum and pericardium,

sternopericardial

_____ ;

pertaining to the sternum and ribs,

sternocostal
(you pronounce)

_____ ;

pertaining to the sternum,

sternal

_____ ;

sternalgia
(you pronounce)

pain in the sternum,

_____ .

58

Stern/o in a word makes you think of the

sternum   _____ which is the

breastbone   _____.

59

Locate the phalanges. They are the ** _____

bones of the
  fingers and toes   _____.

60

phalang   The word root for phalanges is _____.

61

Build a word meaning:

phalang/itis   inflammation of phalanges,
fa lan ji' tis   _____/_____;

phalang/ectomy   excision of one or more phalanges,
fa lan jek' to mi   _____/_____.

62

Locate the acromion. It is a projection of the

shoulder   bone at the _____.

63

The word root-combining form for the acromion

acromi/o   is _____/___.

64

Write a word meaning:

acromi/al   pertaining to the acromion,
acromial
ak ro' mi al   _____/_____;

acromi/o/humer/al   pertaining to the acromion and humerus,
acromiohumeral
a kro' mi o hu mer al   _____/__/_____/_____.

65
Look at the preceding frame. What new word
root-combining form did you use ?

humer/o   _____/___.

66
Humer/o is used in words to refer to the

bone of the upper   ** _____
  arm or humerus
                           _____.

67
Refer back to the drawing of the skeleton. A
condyle is a rounded process that occurs on
many bones. The condyle shown in the draw-

tibia   ing occurs on the _____.

68
Build a word meaning:

                           excision of a condyle,
condyl/ectomy
kon di lek' to mi   _____/_____;

condyl/oid   resembling a condyle,
kon' di loik
                           _____/_____;

epi/condyle   above a condyle,
ep i kon' dil
                           epi /_____;

condyl/ar   pertaining to a condyle,
kon' di lar
                           _____/_____.

69
A ganglion is a collection of nerve cell bodies.
Now that you have a system, form the word
root-combining form for ganglion.

gangli/o   _____/___.

70
Practice identifying the singulars and plurals correctly. Circle the singular noun in each of the following:

ganglion   ganglia/ganglion

acromium   acromia/acromium

ischium   ischii/ischium

calcaneum   calcaneum/calcanea

71
Thromb/o is the word root-combining form that means clot. Thromb/o/angi/itis means inflammation of a vessel with formation of a

clot   _____.

72
Thromb/ectomy means ** _____

excision of a
  thrombus (clot)   _____.

                        Thromb/o/phleb/itis means ** _____

inflammation of a
  vein with thrombus   _____
  formation
                        _____.

73
The proper medical way to say clot is to say

thrombus   thrombus. A synonym for clot is _____.

74
Using thromb/o, build a word meaning:

                        a condition of forming a thrombus,
thromb/osis
throm bo' sis   _____/_____;

thromb/o/cyt/e   a cell that aids in clotting,
throm' bo sit   _____/ / _____/ __;

thromb/oid   resembling a thrombus,
throm boyd'   _____/_____.

75

Phag/o means eat. A phag/o/cyt/e is a cell

eats (or ingests)   that _____ micro-organisms.

76

A macrophage is a large cell that ingests

micr/o/phag/e   micro-organisms. A small cell that ingests
microphage   micro-organisms is called a
mi' kro faj
                         _____ / / _____ / __.

77

What does phagocytosis mean? ** _____

the process of cells   _____
  eating (or ingesting)
  micro-organisms   _____.

Here are 50 more medical terms you have worked with in Unit 9.
Pronounce each aloud; then complete the Unit 9 Self-Test.

acromiohumeral	hemostasis	phalangectomy
ankylocheilia	infracalcaneal	pharyngitis
ankylosis	ischiopubic	pharyngotomy
bacteriostatic	ischiorectal	pleuralgia
bronchitis	laryngeal	pleuritis
bronchoscopy	laryngospasm	pleurocentesis
calcaneal	macrophage	pubic
carpal	microphage	sinistromanual
carpectomy	nasomental	sternal
condyloid	nasopharyngitis	thrombophlebitis
condylectomy	neocyte	thrombosis
dextrocardia	neonatal	tracheorrhagia
dextropedal	neoplasm	tracheotomy
epicondyle	noctambulism	vasoconstriction
fungistasis	noctiphobia	vasospasm
ganglion	nocturia	venostasis
ganglia	phagocytosis	

UNIT 9   SELF-TEST

PART 1

From the list on the right select the correct meaning for each of the following often-used medical terms:

_____ 1. Hemostasis

_____ 2. Pleuralgia

_____ 3. Noctiphobia

_____ 4. Ankylocheilia

_____ 5. Thrombophlebitis

_____ 6. Pleurocentesis

_____ 7. Neoplasm

_____ 8. Ischiopubic

_____ 9. Calcaneal

_____ 10. Dextrocardia

_____ 11. Sinistromanual

_____ 12. Nasomental

_____ 13. Tracheorrhagia

_____ 14. Vasoconstriction

_____ 15. Bacteriostatic

a. Stiffness of the lips

b. Relating to the calcaneus

c. Surgical excision of a condyle

d. Location of the heart on the right

e. A condition of slowing the growth of fungus

f. Slowed blood flow

g. Relating to the ischium and pubis

h. Pertaining to the nose and chin

i. A new growth (tumor)

j. Pain of the pleura

k. Puncture or tapping of the pleura

l. Left-handed

m. Hemorrhage from the trachea

n. Abnormal fear of night (darkness)

o. Inflammation of the vein due to a blood clot

p. Relating to stopping the growth of bacteria

q. Inflammation of the bronchus

r. Constriction of a vessel

PART 2

Write the medical term for each of the following:

1. Spasm of the larynx   _____

2. Inflammation of the pharynx   _____

3. Pertaining to new born   _____

4. Pertaining to the right foot   _____

5. Surgical excision of the carpus   _____

6. Inflammation of the nose and pharynx   _____

7. Relating to the sternum   _____

8. Relating to the pubis   _____

9. Night walking (sleepwalking)   _____

10. Relating to the ischium and rectum   _____

11. Inflammation of the pleura   _____

12. Incision into the trachea   _____

13. Slowing of the flow in the veins   _____

14. Examination by looking into the bronchus   _____

15. Spasm of a vessel   _____

ANSWERS

Part 1

1. f
2. j
3. n
4. a
5. o
6. k
7. i
8. g
9. b
10. d
11. l
12. h
13. m
14. r
15. p

Part 2

1. Laryngospasm
2. Pharyngitis
3. Neonatal
4. Dextropedal
5. Carpectomy
6. Nasopharyngitis
7. Sternal
8. Pubic

9. Noctambulism
10. Ischiorectal
11. Pleuritis
12. Tracheotomy
13. Phlebostasis
14. Bronchoscopy
15. Vasospasm

Unit 10

In this unit you will form more than 80 new medical terms by using what you already know and the following:

core/o, cor/o (pupil)
corne/o (cornea)
cycl/o (ciliary body)
irid/o, ir/o (iris)
kerat/o (cornea)
lacrim/o (tear)
omphal/o (umbilicus, navel)

onych/o (nail)
pod/o (foot)
ren/o (kidney)
retin/o (retina)
scler/o (sclera)
traumat/o (trauma)
tympan/o (eardrum)

Use the following partially labeled drawings of the eye to work the next few frames.

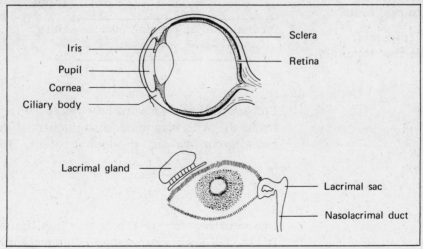

1	
corne/o	The cornea is the transparent layer of tissue covering the iris and pupil. A word root-combining form for cornea is _____/___.

193

2
Write the meaning of each of the following:

inflammation of
  the cornea

corneitis, ** _____

_____;

inflammation of the
  cornea and iris

corneoiritis, ** _____

_____;

the area of the
  cornea and sclera

corneosclera, ** _____

_____.

3
From the preceding frame find two other word
roots that match labels on your drawing. They

ir and scler

are _____ and _____ .

4
The sclera of the eye is the "hard" outer coat
of the eye. Build a word meaning:

scler/al
skle' ra

pertaining to the sclera (adjective),

_____/_____;

scler/ectomy
skle rek' to mi

excision of the sclera (or part),

_____/_____;

scler/ostomy
skle ros' to mi

formation of an opening into the sclera,

_____/_____ .

5
Go back to the other word root you found in
frame 3. With it in mind, find the part of the
eye (on your drawing) to which it refers. This

iris
i' ris

is the _____ .

6
One word root for the iris is ir. It is limited
in use, but always expresses inflammation, so
you can see that it is important.

7

With the information in frame 6 and the word root you found, build a word meaning:

ir/itis

inflammation of the iris, _____/_____;
inflammation of the cornea and iris,

corne/o/ir/itis

_____/____/____/_____;

scler/o/ir/itis
(you pronounce)

inflammation of the sclera and iris,

_____/____/____/_____.

8

Irid/o is the word root-combining form usually used to refer to the iris. Build a word meaning:

irid/o/cele
i rid' o sel

herniation of the iris,

_____/____/_____;

irid/algia
ir id al' ji a

pain in the iris,

_____/_____;

irid/ectomy
ir id ek' to mi

excision of part of the iris,

_____/_____.

9

There are two words to express paralysis of

irid/o/plegia

the iris. They are _____/____/_____

irid/o/paralysis
(you pronounce)

and_____/____/_____.

10

The following forms make you think of:

iris

ir, _____;

iris

irid/o, _____;

sclera (hard)

scler/o, _____;

cornea

corne/o, _____.

11

The word root-combining form for words about

retin/o

the retina is _____/__.

12

Build a word meaning:

retin/al
ret' in al

pertaining to the retina, _____/_____;
inflammation of the retina,

retin/itis
ret in i' tis

_____/_____;

resembling the retina,

retin/oid
ret' in oyd

_____/_____.

13

The instrument used to examine the retina is

retin/o/scop/e
ret' in o skop

the _____/ /_____/____. The
process of examining the retina is

retin/o/scop/y
ret in os' ko pi

_____/ /_____/.

14

The combining form for pupil is cor/e. Build
a word meaning:

cor/ectopia
kor ek to' pi a

pupil misplaced, _____/_____;
destruction of the pupil,

cor/e/lys/is
ko rel' i sis

_____/ /_____/____;

dilatation (stretching) of the pupil,

cor/ectas/ia (is)
kor ek ta' zi a

_____/_____/_____.

15

Core/o is also used as a combining form for
pupil. Using core/o, build a word meaning:

instrument for measuring the pupil,

coreometer

_____;

measurement of the pupil,

coreometry

_____;

plastic surgery of the pupil,

coreoplasty
(you pronounce)

_____.

16

Whether cor/e or core/o is used, the word

cor

root for pupil of the eye is _____.

17

The word root most often used to refer to the cornea is kerat.   Give the combining form:

kerat/o   _____/__.

18

Using kerat/o, build a word meaning:

kerat/ectasia (is)   dilatation of the cornea,
ker a tek ta' si a
                        _____/_____;
kerat/o/plast/y   plastic operation of the cornea (corneal trans-
ker' a to plas ti
                        plant), _____/ /_____/__;
                        incision of the cornea,
kerat/otomy
                        _____/_____;
kerat/o/scler/itis   inflammation of cornea and sclera,
(you pronounce)
                        _____/ /_____/____.

19

Refer to the illustration.   The word root–combining form for ciliary body is cycl/o.   Write a
word meaning:

cycl/o/pleg/ia   paralysis of the ciliary body (noun),
cycloplegia
si klo ple' ji a   _____/ /_____/__;

cycl/o/pleg/ic
cycloplegic   paralysis of the ciliary body (adjective),
si klo ple' jik
                        _____/ /_____/__.

20

Cycloplegia and cycloplegic are words used
often in the specialty of medicine known as

ophthalmology   _____.

21
The following forms make you think of:

retina   retin/o, _____ ;

pupil   cor/e, _____ ;

pupil   core/o, _____ ;

cornea   kerat/o, _____ ;

ciliary body   cycl/o, _____ .

22
Look at the drawing of the lacrimal apparatus.
The word root that you see immediately is

lacrim   _____ . Lacrimal is a word that

tears   means pertaining to _____ .

23
The gland that secretes tears is the

lacrimal
lak' rim al   _____ gland.

24
The sac that collects lacrimal fluid is the

lacrimal   _____ sac.

25
Lacrimal fluid keeps the surface of the eye
moistened. It is continually forming and being
removed. When there is more formed than
can be removed by the apparatus, you say the

crying or tearing   person is ** _____ .

26
Give a word meaning instrument for incising the:

keratotome
ker at' o tom   cornea, _____ ;

sclerotome
skler' o tom   sclera, _____ .

27

The two combining forms used in building the

phag/o   word phagocyte are _____ / ___ and

cyt/o   _____ / ___ .

28

Phag/o is a combining form meaning eat. The
word phag/o/cyt/e makes you think literally of

eats (or   a cell that _____ .
 ingests)

29

A phagocyte ingests (absorbs, eats--after a
fashion) other cells, bacteria, or waste matter.

embryonic phago-   A phagocytoblast is an ** _____
 cyte or a cell that
 will become a   _____
 phagocyte
                    _____ .

30

Phagocytosis is the condition of absorption or

phagocytes   digestion by _____ .

31

Cyt/o/phag/o/cyt/osis is ** _____

the ingestion (des-   _____
 truction or eating)
 of cells by   _____
 phagocytes
                       _____ .

32

                An instrument for measuring cells is a

cyt/o/meter
si tom' et er   _____ / ___ / _____ . The process of

cyt/o/metry
si tom' et ry   measuring cells is _____ / ___ / _____ .

The next five frames will give you more practice in finding word root-combining forms.
New words enter the medical vocabulary constantly.

33

The tympanum is the eardrum. The word
root-combining form for tympanum is

tympan/o   _____/____. Write a word that means
surgical repair of the eardrum:

tympanoplasty   _____.

34

Build a word meaning:

tympan/ic (al)   pertaining to the eardrum,
tympanic
tim pan' ik   _____/_____;

tympan/otomy   incision into the eardrum,
tympanotomy
tim pan ot' o mi   _____/_____;

tympan/ectomy   excision of the eardrum,
tympanectomy
tim pan ek' to mi   _____/_____.

35

ren/al   Ren/o is the word root-combining form used
renal   for kidney. Build a word meaning:
re' nal   pertaining to the kidney, _____/_____;
                         record from x-ray of the kidney,
ren/o/graph (gram)
(you pronounce)   _____/ /_____.

36

                         Renointestinal means ** _____
pertaining to the
  kidney and intestine   _____.

                         Renogastric means ** _____
pertaining to the
  kidney and stomach   _____.

37

Pod/o refers to the foot. Build a word meaning:

pod/algia   foot pain, _____/_____;

pod/o/gram   footprint, _____/___/ gram .

38

A review. Crypt/orchi/ism is the condition or state of having undescended testes. Hyper/

condition or state   thyroid/ism is a ** _____
 of too much
 secretion by the   _____
 thyroid gland
                         _____.

39

condition or state   Hypo/pituitar/ism is a ** _____
 of too little secre-
 tion of the pituitary   _____
 gland
                         _____.

40

A psychiatrist practices psychiatry. One whose practice of medicine is limited to diseases of

ophthalmologist   the eye is an _____.

41

                         The suffix emia means ** _____
condition of blood
 or blood condition   _____.

42

Isch/emia is a condition in which blood is drained from one place. A condition of too
leuk/emia   many leukocytes in the blood is called
leukemia
lu ke' mi a   _____/_____.

an/emia
an e' mi a

hyper/emia
hi per e' mi a

ur/emia
u re' mi a

43
Build a word meaning:

without (not enough) blood, _____/_____ ;
too much blood (in one part),

_____/_____ :

urine constituents in blood,

_____/_____ .

yellow color
   in the blood

redness of the
   blood (blushing)

44
Write a meaning for

xanthemia, ** _____

_____ ;

erythremia, ** _____

_____ .

umbilicus

45
To find a word root for the navel look up navel
in your dictionary. A synonym for navel is

_____ .

navel

46
The word root-combining form for umbilicus
is omphal/o. Words beginning with omphal/o
refer to the umbilicus, also called the

_____ .

omphal/ic
om fal' ik

omphal/ectomy
om fal ek' to mi

omphal/o/cele
om fal' o sel

47
Using omphal/o, build a word meaning:

pertaining to the navel, _____/____ ;
excision of the umbilicus,

_____/_____ ;

herniation of the navel,

_____/__/_____ .

48
Build a word meaning:

umbilical hemorrhage,

omphal/orrhagia   _____/_____;

discharge flowing from the navel,

omphal/orrhea   _____/_____;

omphalorrhexis   rupture of the navel,
(you pronounce)   _____/_____.

49
Words containing omphal/o refer to the

navel   _____, which is also called the

umbilicus   _____.

50
A word root for nail is onych. The word root-
combining form that refers to nail is

onych/o   _____/__.

51
Build a word meaning:

resembling a finger nail,

onych/oid   _____/_____;
on' i koyd
                       tumor of the nail (or nail bed),
onych/oma
on i ko' ma   _____/_____;

onych/osis   any nail condition,
on i ko' sis   _____/_____.

52
What does paronychia mean? ** _____

a condition (usually   _____
  inflammation)
  around the nails   _____.

53
Give a meaning for onychocryptosis:

literally a condition
of a nail being
hidden or ingrown
toenail

** _____

_____

_____ .

You now know a good system for word building. You know many prefixes, suffixes, and combining forms from singular and plural forms of a word. You also know several ways to find combining forms in your dictionary.

54
To prove it again look up trauma in your dictionary. It means ** _____

a wound or
injury

_____ . Write the plural form:

traumata

_____ .

55
The combining form is derived from the plural

traumat/o

form and is _____ / __ .

56
A word meaning referring to injury or of injury

traumatic

is _____ .

traumat/o/log/y
traumatology
traw ma tol' o ji

The study of caring for wounds is called

_____ / __ / _____ / __ .

Here are fifty of the medical terms you worked with in Unit 10.
Don't forget to pronounce each one carefully before taking the final
Unit 10 Self-Test.

corectasia	keratectasia	retinitis
corectopia	keratome	retinoid
corelysis	keratoplasty	retinoscopy
coreometer	keratoscleritis	sclerectomy
coreoplasty	keratotomy	scleroiritis
corneal	lacrimal	sclerotome
corneitis	nasolacrimal	traumata
corneoiritis	omphalorrhexis	traumatic
corneosclera	omphalic	traumatology
cycloplegia	onychocryptosis	tympanic
cycloplegic	onychoid	tympanectomy
iridalgia	onychoma	tympanoplasty
iridectomy	ophthalmologist	tympanorrhaphy
iridocele	podalgia	tympanotomy
iridoparalysis	podogram	tympanum
iridoplegia	renogram	uremia
iritis	renointestinal	

UNIT 10   SELF-TEST

PART 1

From the list on the right, select the correct meaning for each of the following medical terms:

_____ 1. Renogram

_____ 2. Onychoid

_____ 3. Tympanorrhaphy

_____ 4. Keratoscleritis

_____ 5. Traumatology

_____ 6. Corectasia

_____ 7. Corneosclera

_____ 8. Ophthalmologist

_____ 9. Iridoplegia

_____ 10. Corneal

_____ 11. Omphalorrhexis

_____ 12. Keratome

_____ 13. Iridocele

_____ 14. Retinoid

_____ 15. Onychocryptosis

a. Stretching (dilatation) of the pupil

b. Relating to the cornea

c. Inflammation of the sclera and iris

d. The membrane that forms the cornea and sclera

e. Painful foot

f. Herniation of the iris

g. Paralysis of the iris

h. Instrument to cut the cornea

i. Inflammation of the cornea and sclera

j. Rupture of the umbilicus

k. Condition of hidden nail (ingrown nail)

l. Resembling a nail

m. A physician who specializes in the study of eye diseases

n. Picture (x-ray) of the kidney

o. Resembling the retina

p. Instrument to cut the sclera

q. The scientific study of trauma

r. Suturing of the eardrum

PART 2

Write the medical term for each of the following:

1. Surgical repair (plastic surgery of) the tympanum _____

2. Instrument for measuring the pupil _____

3. Relating to trauma _____

4. Inflammation of the cornea and iris _____

5. Surgical removal of the sclera _____

6. Paralysis of the ciliary body   Cyclo _____

7. Examination of the retina (looking at) _____

8. Surgical excision of the iris _____

9. Inflammation of the retina _____

10. Paralysis of the iris _____

11. Footprint _____

12. Dilatation (stretching) of the cornea   Kerat _____

13. Incision into the cornea _____

14. Inflammation of the iris _____

15. Relating to the nose and lacrimal duct _____

ANSWERS

Part 1

1.	n	9.	g
2.	l	10.	b
3.	r	11.	j
4.	i	12.	h
5.	q	13.	f
6.	a	14.	o
7.	d	15.	k
8.	m		

Part 2

1. Tympanoplasty
2. Coreometer
3. Traumatic
4. Corneoiritis
5. Sclerectomy
6. Cycloplegia
7. Retinoscopy
8. Iridectomy
9. Retinitis
10. Iridoplegia or iridoparalysis
11. Podogram
12. Keratectasia
13. Keratotomy
14. Iritis
15. Nasolacrimal or rhinolacrimal

Review Sheets

Following are review sheets for each unit, which will be useful not only as you are working through QUICK MEDICAL TERMINOLOGY but also as a refresher later on. You should rework these review sheets whenever word parts begin to fade in your memory. Of course, the more practice you have, the better you will know the material.

Answers are given on the right; as before, you may wish to cover the answer column with a piece of paper while you work the review sheet. For further reference the glossary of word parts will tell you where each part was introduced.

UNIT 1: REVIEW SHEET

Part 1

WORD PART	MEANING	
acr/o	_____	extremity
megal/o	_____	enlargement
dermat/o	_____	skin
cyan/o	_____	blue
derm/o	_____	skin
leuk/o	_____	white
itis	_____	inflammation
cardi/o	_____	heart
gastr/o	_____	stomach
cyt/o	_____	cell
ologist	_____	one who studies
algia	_____	pain
ectomy	_____	excision
otomy	_____	incision
ostomy	_____	new opening
duoden/o	_____	duodenum
electr/o	_____	electricity
ology	_____	study of
osis	_____	condition of
tome	_____	instrument that cuts
gram/o	_____	record

Part 2

MEANING	WORD PART	
record	_____	gram/o
one who studies	_____	ologist
enlargement	_____	megal/o
electricity	_____	electr/o
white	_____	leuk/o
incision	_____	otomy
blue	_____	cyan/o
instrument that cuts	_____	tome
stomach	_____	gastr/o
extremity	_____	acr/o
condition of	_____	osis
new opening	_____	ostomy
skin	_____	dermat/o, derm/o
study of	_____	ology
heart	_____	cardi/o
excision	_____	ectomy
inflammation	_____	itis
duodenum	_____	duoden/o
pain	_____	algia
cell	_____	cyt/o

UNIT 2: REVIEW SHEET

Part 1

WORD PART	MEANING	
aden/o	_____	gland
carcin/o	_____	cancer
malac/o	_____	softening
oid	_____	resembling
laryng/o	_____	larynx
cephal/o	_____	head
hyper	_____	over, more than normal
cele	_____	herniation
oste/o	_____	bone
arthr/o	_____	joint
chondr/o	_____	cartilage
cost/o	_____	rib
lip/o	_____	fat
inter	_____	between
dent/o	_____	tooth
emesis	_____	vomiting
inter	_____	between
oma	_____	tumor
plast/o, plast/y	_____	repair
hypo	_____	under, less than normal
troph/o	_____	development

Part 2

MEANING	WORD PART	
rib	_____	cost/o
larynx	_____	laryng/o
development	_____	troph/o
cancer	_____	carcin/o
repair	_____	plast/o (/y)
tooth	_____	dent/o
mucus	_____	muc/o
under, less than normal	_____	hypo
herniation	_____	cele
softening	_____	malac/o
gland	_____	aden/o
water	_____	hydr/o
tumor	_____	oma
bone	_____	oste/o
vomiting	_____	emesis
head	_____	cephal/o
joint	_____	arthr/o
between	_____	inter
resembling	_____	oid
fat	_____	lip/o
between	_____	inter
cartilage	_____	chondr/o
over, more than normal	_____	hyper

UNIT 3: REVIEW SHEET

Part 1

WORD PART	MEANING
cyst/o	_____ bladder
supra	_____ above
crani/o	_____ cranium (skull)
pub/o	_____ pubis
cerebr/o	_____ cerebrum
ab	_____ away from
cocc/i	_____ coccus
metr/o, meter	_____ measure
py/o	_____ pus
genesis, gen/o	_____ formation, development
orrhea	_____ flow
ot/o	_____ ear
centesis	_____ puncture
rhin/o	_____ nose
lith/o	_____ stone or calculus
hydr/o	_____ water
chol/e	_____ gall, bile
scope, scopy	_____ examining
thorac/o	_____ thorax or chest
pelv/i	_____ pelvis
cyst/o	_____ bladder
ad	_____ toward
abdomin/o	_____ abdomen
therap/o	_____ treatment
lumb/o	_____ loin
phob/ia	_____ fear

Part 2

MEANING	WORD PART	
water	_____	hydr/o
flow	_____	orrhea
fear	_____	phob/ia
pubis	_____	pub/o
loin	_____	lumb/o
pelvis	_____	pelv/i
gall, bile	_____	chol/e
nose	_____	rhin/o
puncture	_____	centesis
cerebrum	_____	cerebr/o
pus	_____	py/o
treatment	_____	therap/o
toward	_____	ad
formation, development	_____	genesis, gen/o
above	_____	supra
bladder	_____	cyst/o
coccus	_____	cocc/i
measure	_____	metr/o, meter
examining	_____	scope, scopy
stone or calculus	_____	lith/o
ear	_____	ot/o
breathe	_____	pne/o
thorax or chest	_____	thorac/o
cranium (skull)	_____	crani/o
bladder	_____	cyst/o
softening	_____	malac/o
away from	_____	ab
abdomen	_____	abdomin/o

Part 3

Suffixes that make a word an adjective meaning pertaining to:

SUFFIXES	EXAMPLE
al	duoden/al
ic	gastr/ic
ar	lumb/ar
ac	cardi/ac

Prepare a list of word roots using these adjective endings.   Add to this list as you learn new words.

al   ic   ar   ac

UNIT 4: REVIEW SHEET

Part 1

WORD PART	MEANING	
peps/ia	_____	digestion
neur/o	_____	nerve
blast/o	_____	embryonic form
a, an	_____	without
angi/o	_____	vessel
spasm	_____	twitching
scler/o	_____	hard
tachy	_____	fast
my/o	_____	muscle
fibr/o	_____	fibrous, fiber
lys/o	_____	destruction
pne/o	_____	breathe
arteri/o	_____	artery
hem/o	_____	blood
hemat/o	_____	blood
kinesi/o	_____	movement
spermat/o	_____	spermatozoa
oophor/o	_____	ovary
pexe/o (/y)	_____	fixation
salping/o	_____	fallopian tube
dys	_____	bad, painful, difficult
hyster/o	_____	uterus
ptosis	_____	prolapse, drooping
brady	_____	slow
ur/o	_____	urine
blephar/o	_____	eyelid

nephr/o _____ kidney

pyel/o _____ renal pelvis

ureter/o _____ ureter

orrhaphy _____ suture

urethr/o _____ urethra

orrhagia _____ hemorrhage

pneumon/o _____ lung

pneum/o _____ lung

pne/o _____ breathing

melan/o _____ black

Part 2

MEANING	WORD PART	
artery	_____	arteri/o
vessel	_____	angi/o
uterus	_____	hyster/o
movement	_____	kinesi/o
destruction	_____	lys/o
blood	_____	hemat/o, hem/o
blood	_____	hem/o, hemat/o
urine	_____	ur/o
hard	_____	scler/o
slow	_____	brady
fallopian tube	_____	salping/o
muscle	_____	my/o
without	_____	a, an
nerve	_____	neur/o
fixation	_____	pex/y (/y)
embryonic form	_____	blast/o

ovary	_____	oophor/o
breathe	_____	pne/o
digestion	_____	peps/ia
prolapse, drooping	_____	ptosis
bad, painful, difficult	_____	dys
spermatozoa	_____	spermat/o
fibrous, fiber	_____	fibr/o
twitching	_____	spasm
fast	_____	tachy
hemorrhage	_____	orrhagia
renal pelvis	_____	pyel/o
black	_____	melan/o
ureter	_____	ureter/o
kidney	_____	nephr/o
lung	_____	pneumon/o
lung	_____	pneum/o
urethra	_____	urethr/o
suture	_____	orrhaphy
breathing	_____	pne/o
eyelid	_____	blephar/o

UNIT 5: REVIEW SHEET

Part 1

WORD PART	MEANING	
stomat/o	_____	mouth
gloss/o	_____	tongue
cheil/o	_____	lips
gingiv/o	_____	gums
esophag/o	_____	esophagus
enter/o	_____	small intestine
col/o	_____	colon
rect/o	_____	rectum
proct/o	_____	anus or rectum
hepat/o	_____	liver
pancreat/o	_____	pancreas
clys/o, -clys/is	_____	wash, irrigate
ectasia	_____	dilatation, stretch
pleg/a (/ia, /ic)	_____	paralysis
phleb/o	_____	vein
my/o	_____	muscle
orrhexis	_____	rupture
esthesia	_____	feeling, sensation
algesia	_____	abnormal sensitivity
phas/o	_____	speech
dipl/o	_____	double
opia	_____	vision
tripsy	_____	surgical crushing
plas/o	_____	formation, development

psych/o	_____	mind or soul
pro	_____	before
gnosis	_____	knowledge or know
di/a	_____	through
orrhexis	_____	rupture

Part 2

MEANING	WORD PART	
paralysis	_____	pleg/a (/ia, /ic)
liver	_____	hepat/o
muscle	_____	my/o
small intestine	_____	enter/o
feeling, sensation	_____	esthesia
speech	_____	phas/o
abnormal sensitivity	_____	algesia
anus or rectum	_____	proct/o
lips	_____	cheil/o
wash, irrigate	_____	clys/is, clys/o
esophagus	_____	esophag/o
colon	_____	col/o
gums	_____	gingiv/o
mouth	_____	stomat/o
vein	_____	phleb/o
dilatation, stretch	_____	ectasia
pancreas	_____	pancreat/o
rectum	_____	rect/o
tongue	_____	gloss/o
rupture	_____	orrhexis

formation, development	_____	plas/o
double	_____	dipl/o
rupture	_____	orrhexis
mind or soul	_____	psych/o
through	_____	di/a
surgical crushing	_____	trips/y
before	_____	pro
vision	_____	opia
knowledge or know	_____	gnosis
heat	_____	therm/o
small	_____	micr/o
large	_____	macr/o
bone marrow, spinal cord	_____	myel/o
finger or toe	_____	dactyl/o
many	_____	pol/y
with, together	_____	syn
running with, symptom	_____	drom/o

UNIT 6: REVIEW SHEET

Part 1

WORD PART	MEANING
anter/o	_____ before
poster/o	_____ behind, after
dors/o	_____ back
ventr/o	_____ belly
caud/o	_____ tail
men/o	_____ menses, menstruation
stasis	_____ halt, control
syphil/o	_____ syphilis
lapar/o	_____ abdominal wall
pyr/o	_____ fever, fire
xanth/o	_____ yellow
chlor/o	_____ green
erythr/o	_____ red
derm/o	_____ skin
emia	_____ blood
hidr/o	_____ sweat
gynec/o	_____ woman
ophthalm/o	_____ eye
viscer/o	_____ internal organs
later/o	_____ side

Part 2

MEANING	WORD PART	
back	_____	dors/o
tail	_____	caud/o
menses, menstruation	_____	men/o
syphilis	_____	syphil/o
belly	_____	ventr/o
before	_____	anter/o
halt, control	_____	stasis
behind, after	_____	poster/o
skin	_____	derm/o
yellow	_____	xanth/o
side	_____	later/o
internal organs	_____	viscer/o
sweat	_____	hidr/o
abdominal wall	_____	lapar/o
eye	_____	ophthalm/o
fever, fire	_____	pyr/o
woman	_____	gynec/o
red	_____	erythr/o
blood	_____	emia, hemat/o, hem/o
green	_____	chlor/o

UNIT 7: REVIEW SHEET

Part 1

WORD PART	MEANING	
orchid/o	_____	testes, testicles
crypt/o	_____	hidden
colp/o	_____	vagina
end/o	_____	inner
mes/o	_____	middle
ect/o	_____	outer
ectopic	_____	misplaced
retr/o	_____	behind, backward
par/a	_____	around
aut/o	_____	self
mon/o	_____	single
mult/i	_____	many
glyc/o	_____	sugar
heter/o	_____	different
par/o	_____	bear
splen/o	_____	spleen
sym	_____	together
null/i	_____	none
ab	_____	from, away from
ad	_____	toward
de	_____	from, down from
ex	_____	from, out from
narc/o	_____	sleep
leps/o	_____	seizure
is/o	_____	equal
peri	_____	around

circum   _____   around

di/a   _____   through

per   _____   through

necr/o   _____   dead

phil/o   _____   attraction

hom/o   _____   same

super   _____   beyond

supra   _____   above

Part 2

MEANING	WORD PART
spleen	_____ splen/o
outer, outside	_____ ect/o
bear	_____ par/o
many	_____ mult/i
testes, testicles	_____ orchid/o
inner	_____ end/o
behind, backward	_____ retr/o
sugar	_____ glyc/o
together	_____ syn, sym
middle	_____ mes/o
single	_____ mon/o
around	_____ par/a
hidden	_____ crypt/o
misplaced	_____ ectopic
vagina	_____ colp/o
different	_____ heter/o
sleep	_____ narc/o
attraction	_____ phil/o
out from	_____ ex

away from	_____	ab
down from	_____	de
toward	_____	ad
none	_____	null/i
same	_____	hom/o
seizure	_____	leps/o
dead	_____	necr/o
equal	_____	is/o
through	_____	per, di/a
around	_____	circum, peri, para
above	_____	supra
beyond	_____	super

UNIT 8: REVIEW SHEET

Part 1

WORD PART	MEANING
semi	_____ half
metr/o, hyster/o	_____ uterus
uni	_____ one
mal	_____ bad, poor
epi	_____ over, upon
extra	_____ in addition to, outside of
infra	_____ under, below
sub	_____ under, below
post	_____ behind, after
dis	_____ free of
anti	_____ against
contra	_____ against
trans	_____ across, over
sanguin/o	_____ blood relationship
ante	_____ before, forward
bi	_____ two, double
con	_____ with
hemi	_____ half
pre	_____ before, in front of
tri	_____ three
intr/a	_____ within

Part 2

MEANING	WORD PART	
with	_____	con
in addition to, outside of	_____	extra
free of	_____	dis
against	_____	contra, anti
behind, after	_____	post
across, over	_____	trans
one	_____	uni, mono
under, below	_____	sub, infra
within	_____	intr/a, in
over, upon	_____	epi
uterus	_____	hyster/o, metr/o
two, double	_____	bi
half	_____	hemi, semi
bad, poor	_____	mal
before, forward	_____	ante
before, in front of	_____	pre
three	_____	tri
blood relationship	_____	sanguin/o

UNIT 9: REVIEW SHEET

Part 1

WORD PART	MEANING	
nas/o	_____	nose
pharyng/o	_____	pharynx
laryng/o	_____	larynx
trache/o	_____	trachea
bronch/o	_____	bronchus
pleur/o	_____	pleura
sinistr/o	_____	left
dextr/o	_____	right
vas/o	_____	vessel
ne/o	_____	new
ment/o	_____	chin
phag/o	_____	eat
noct/i	_____	night
ankyl/o	_____	stiff
calcane/o	_____	heel
pharyng/o	_____	pharynx
carp/o	_____	wrist
ischi/o	_____	ischium
stern/o	_____	sternum, breastbone
phalang/o	_____	bones of fingers and toes
acromi/o	_____	acromion
humer/o	_____	humerus
condyl/o	_____	condyle
gangli/o	_____	ganglion
thromb/o	_____	clot, thrombus

plasm   _____   formation

manual   _____   -handed

pedal   _____   -footed

Part 2

MEANING	WORD PART	
eat	_____	phag/o
nose	_____	nas/o, rhin/o
pleura	_____	pleur/o
larynx	_____	laryng/o
chin	_____	ment/o
right	_____	dextr/o
bronchus	_____	bronch/o
vessel	_____	vas/o
left	_____	sinistr/o
trachea	_____	trache/o
new	_____	ne/o
pharynx	_____	pharyng/o
-handed	_____	manual
-footed	_____	pedal
night	_____	noct/i
wrist	_____	carp/o
formation	_____	plasm, plas/o, troph/o, gen/o
clot, thrombus	_____	thromb/o
humerus	_____	humer/o
heel	_____	calcane/o
sternum, breastbone	_____	stern/o
ganglion	_____	gangli/o
ischium	_____	ischi/o

condyle _____ condyl/o

acromion _____ acromi/o

pharynx _____ pharyng/o

bones of fingers
  and toes _____ phalang/o

stiff _____ ankyl/o

UNIT 10: REVIEW SHEET

Part 1

WORD PART	MEANING	
corne/o	_____	cornea
scler/o	_____	sclera
ir/o	_____	iris
irid/o	_____	iris
retin/o	_____	retina
cor/o, core/o	_____	pupil
kerat/o	_____	cornea
cycl/o	_____	ciliary body
lacrim/o	_____	tear
tympan/o	_____	eardrum
ren/o	_____	kidney
pod/o	_____	foot
omphal/o	_____	navel, umbilicus
onych/o	_____	nail
traumat/o	_____	trauma
phag/o	_____	eat

Part 2

MEANING	WORD PART
cornea	_____	kerat/o, corne/o
cornea	_____	corne/o, kerat/o
iris	_____	ir/o, irid/o
retina	_____	retin/o
tear	_____	lacrim/o
nail	_____	onych/o
eardrum	_____	tympan/o
navel	_____	omphal/o
ciliary body	_____	cycl/o
sclera	_____	scler/o
foot	_____	pod/o
kidney	_____	ren/o
pupil	_____	cor/o, core/o
trauma	_____	.traumat/o
eat	_____	phag/o

Final Self-Test I

INSTRUCTIONS

The following two tests will show you how much you have learned about medical terminology. Many of the words on the tests will be new to you; however, using the word parts and the word-building system you have learned, you should be able to give the meaning for all of them. Try these tests and see how well you do. You may want to take one test before reading the book and the other after you finish the book. That will show even more clearly how much medical terminology you have learned.

Each test consists of 50 medical terms. For each term write out a definition in your own words. Then compare your answers with those following the test. Your definition should include all of the ideas (though not necessarily in the exact words) as the definitions on the answer page.

TEST 1

1. Tachypnea _____

2. Oophoritis _____

3. Pyelonephrosis _____

4. Acroparalysis _____

5. Bradypepsia _____

6. Glycolysis _____

7. Blepharospasm _____

8. Megalocardia _____

9. Ophthalmoscopy _____

10. Bronchopneumonogram _____

11. Hemiplegia _____

12. Uterocele _____

13. Cephalometer _____

14. Antispasmodic _____

15. Hyperthyroidism _____

16. Bronchiectasis _____

17. Aphagia _____

18. Xanthemia _____

19. Symptomatology _____

20. Rhinologist _____

21. Kinesiology _____

22. Fibroosteoma _____

23. Anuria _____

24. Lipochondroma _____

25. Costectomy _____

26. Polyotia _____

27. Tracheorrhagia _____

28. Paranephritis _____

29. Enteroptosis _____

30. Erythrocyte _____

31. Perianal _____

32. Endocarditis _____

33. Lymphadenoid _____

34. Thoracolumbar _____

35. Corneoiritis _____

36. Hepatorrhexis _____

37. Thrombogenesis _____

38. Hematoma _____

39. Lithotomy _____

40. Rectorrhaphy _____

41. Cardiac hypertrophy _____

42. Phleboplasty _____

43. Dorsalgia _____

44. Endocranial _____

45. Cardiotomy _____

46. Adenocarcinoma _____

47. Esophagogastrostomy _____

48. Enterohepatitis _____

49. Arteriosclerosis _____

50. Dyspeptic _____

ANSWERS TO FINAL SELF-TEST I

1. rapid breathing
2. inflammation of an ovary
3. condition (abnormal or diseased) of the pelvis of the kidney
4. paralysis of the extremities
5. slow digestion
6. destruction (breakdown) of sugar (glucose)
7. spasm (twitching) of the eyelid
8. excessively large heart
9. examination of the interior of the eye
10. record (picture) of the bronchi and lungs
11. paralysis of one half (one side) of the body
12. hernia of the uterus
13. instrument for measuring the head
14. a substance that relieves or checks spasms
15. a condition caused by excessive secretion of the thyroid glands
16. dilatation of the bronchi
17. inability to swallow (eat)
18. yellow pigment (color) in the blood
19. the study (science) of disease symptoms
20. a specialist in diseases of the nose
21. the study (science) of muscular movement
22. a tumor of bone and fibrous tissue
23. absence of urine
24. a tumor of cartilaginous and fatty tissue
25. excision of a rib or ribs
26. the state of having more than two ears
27. hemorrhage within the trachea
28. inflammation of tissues around (surrounding) the kidney
29. sagging of the intestine
30. red blood cell
31. of or pertaining to around the anus
32. inflammation of the inside (lining) of the heart
33. resembling the lymph glands
34. of or pertaining to the chest (thorax) and lower back (lumbar)
35. inflammation of the iris and cornea
36. rupture of the liver
37. formation (development) of a clot (thrombus)
38. blood tumor (bruise)
39. surgical removal of a stone (calculus)
40. suturing (stitching) of the rectum
41. a condition of excessive enlargement of the heart
42. surgical repair of a vein
43. pain in the back
44. of or pertaining to the inside of the head
45. surgical incision of the heart
46. malignant tumor of a gland
47. making a new opening (permanent) between the esophagus and the stomach
48. inflammation of the liver and intestine
49. a condition of hardening of the arteries
50. of or pertaining to painful digestion

Final Self-Test II

1. Uremia _____
2. Acidosis _____
3. Amenorrhea _____
4. Antipyretic _____
5. Nephrolith _____
6. Enterectasia _____
7. Acardiohemia _____
8. Encephalorrhagia _____
9. Craniocele _____
10. Blepharoptosis _____
11. Gastroparalysis _____
12. Cholecystitis _____
13. Abdominalgia _____
14. Arteriospasm _____
15. Adenosclerosis _____
16. Duodenohepatic _____
17. Endobronchitis _____
18. Iridomalacia _____
19. Duodeno-enterostomy _____
20. Megalogastria _____
21. Phleborrhexis _____

22. Microscope _____

23. Osteoid _____

24. Electroencephalogram _____

25. Hepatoma _____

26. Hemotherapy _____

27. Intercostal _____

28. Dyspneic _____

29. Urethrocystitis _____

30. Hypothyroidism _____

31. Traumatology _____

32. Pericardiectomy _____

33. Syndrome _____

34. Hepatorrhaphy _____

35. Adhesiotomy _____

36. Nephropexy _____

37. Pneumonomelanosis _____

38. Cerebrovascular _____

39. Chondromalacia _____

40. Intravenous _____

41. Periosteal _____

42. Leukocytolysis _____

43. Salpingostomy _____

44. Paraproctitis _____

45. Kinesthetic _____

46. Xanthoderma _____

47. Ophthalmoplegia _____

48. Hydrothorax _____

49. Otorhinolaryngologist _____

50. Suprapubic _____

ANSWERS TO FINAL SELF-TEST II

1. excessive urine in the blood
2. a condition of excess acid in the body
3. cessation of menstruation
4. a substance that counteracts (acts against) the effects of a fever
5. a stone (calculus) in the kidney
6. dilatation of the small intestine
7. insufficient blood in the heart
8. hemorrhage within the brain
9. hernia of structures in the skull (cranium)
10. drooping (prolapse) of the eyelids
11. paralysis of the stomach
12. inflammation of the gall bladder
13. painful abdomen
14. spasm (twitching) of an artery
15. a condition of hardening of glandular tissue
16. of or pertaining to the duodenum and liver
17. inflammation of the inside of the bronchi
18. softening of the iris
19. making a new permanent opening between the duodenum and the small intestine
20. excessively large stomach
21. rupture of a vein
22. an instrument for examing very small units
23. resembling bone
24. a record (picture) of electrical activity in the brain
25. tumor of the liver
26. the use of blood (transfusion) in treating diseases
27. between the ribs
28. of or pertaining to painful breathing
29. inflammation of the urethra and bladder
30. a condition of insufficient thyroid excretion
31. the study (science) of injuries and their effect on the body
32. excision of tissue around the heart
33. a group of symptoms occurring together
34. suturing (stitching) the liver
35. surgical incision of adhesions
36. surgical fixation of the kidney
37. a condition of black lungs
38. of or pertaining to the vessels of the brain
39. softening (wasting) of cartilage tissue
40. within a vein
41. of or pertaining to tissues surrounding the bone
42. destruction of white blood cells
43. surgical opening into a fallopian tube
44. inflammation of tissues surrounding the anus and rectum
45. of or pertaining to the sensation of movement
46. skin of yellow color
47. paralysis of the eye
48. water in the chest cavity
49. a specialist in ear, nose, and throat diseases
50. of or pertaining to the area above the pubis

Glossary of Word Parts Learned

The following word parts are listed by page number.

a, 58
ab, 37
abdomin/o, 38
acr/o, 6
acromi/o, 186
ad, 36
aden/o, 23
alges/i, 93
algia, 13
an, 92
angi/o, 60
ankyl/o, 180
ante, 163
anter/o, 110
anti, 154
appendic/o, 167
arteri/o, 61
arthr/o, 29
aut/o, 132
bi, 159
blast/o, 60
blephar/o, 69
brad/y, 55
bronch/o (/i), 175
calcane/o, 183
carcin/o, 24
cardi/o, 11
carp/o, 183
caud/o, 110
cele, 28
centesis, 38
cephal/o, 26

cerebr/o, 43
cheil/o, 81
chlor/o, 114
chol/e, 48
chondr/o, 30
circum, 138
clysis, 86
cocc/o, 44
col/o, 87
colp/o, 127
con, 161
condyl/o, 187
contra, 155
cor/o, core/o, 196
corne/o, 193
cortic/o, 167
cost/o, 31
crani/o, 43
crypt/o, 127
cyan/o, 8
cycl/o, 197
cyst/o, 38
cyt/o, 10
dactyl/o, 102
de, 135
dent/o, 31
derm/o, 10
dermat/o, 7
dextr/o, 177
di/a, 99
dipl/o, 95
dis, 162

dors/o, 110
drom/o, 104
duoden/o, 14
dys, 59
ect/o, 128
ectas/ia (/is), 86
ectomy, 14
ectopic, 130
electr/o, 13
emesis, 22
emia, 116
encephal/o, 27
end/o, 128
enter/o, 81
epi, 152
erythr/o, 114
esophag/o, 90
esthesi/o, 92
ex, 136
extra, 152
femor/o, 185
fibr/o, 61
gangli/o, 187
gastr/o, 12
genesis, 45
gingiv/o, 85
gloss/o, 83
glyc/o, 125
gnos/o, 99
gram/o, 13
graph/o, 13
gynec/o, 117

hem/o, 62
hemat/o, 62
hemi, 160
hepat/o, 89
heter/o, 142
hidr/o, 116
hom/o, 142
humer/o, 186
hydr/o, 40
hyper, 21
hypo, 22
hyster/o, 68
in, 157
infra, 153
inter, 31
intr/a, 164
ir/o, 194
irid/o, 195
is/o, 137
ischi/o, 184
itis, 8
kerat/o, 197
kinesi/o, 56
lacrim/o, 198
lapar/o, 113
laryng/o, 25
later/o, 111
leps/o, 137
leuk/o, 10
lip/o, 24
lith/o, 47
log/o, 12
lumb/o, 41
lys/o, 60
macr/o, 101
mal, 158
malac/o, 28
manual, 177
medi/o, 111
megal/o, 7
melan/o, 75
men/o, 111
mes/o, 128
metr/o, meter, 43
metr/o (uterus), 150

micr/o, 101
mon/o, 132
muc/o, 25
mult/i, 132
my/o, 94
myel/o, 96
narc/o, 136
nas/o, 173
necr/o, 140
ne/o, 179
nephr/o, 69
neur/o, 60
noct/i, 179
null/i, 133
o/o, 64
oid, 24
oma, 23
omphal/o, 202
onych/o, 203
oophor/o, 65
ophthalm/o, 117
opia, 95
orchid/o, 126
orrhagia, 73
orrhaphy, 72
orrhea, 45
orrhexis, 91
osis, 8
oste/o, 29
ostomy, 15
ot/o, 46
otomy, 15
pancreat/o, 89
par/a, 131
par/o, 133
pedal, 177
pelv/i, 42
peps/o, 59
per, 139
peri, 138
pex/o, 65
phag/o, 189
phalang/o, 186
pharyng/o, 174
phas/o, 93

phil/o, 141
phleb/o, 91
phob/o, 40
plas/o, 97
plasm, 179
plast/o, 29
pleg/a, 81
pleur/o, 176
pne/o, 57
pneum/o, 74
pneumon/o, 74
pod/o, 201
pol/y, 102
post, 163
poster/o, 110
pre, 163
pro, 99
proct/o, 88
psych/o, 97
ptosis, 68
pub/o, 42
py/o, 45
pyel/o, 71
pyr/o, 114
rect/o, 87
ren/o, 200
retin/o, 195
retr/o, 130
rhin/o, 47
salping/o, 66
sanguin/o, 161
scler/o, 61
scop/o, 81
semi, 160
sinistr/o, 176
spasm, 60
spermat/o, 63
splen/o, 143
staphyl/o, 44
stasis, 112
stern/o, 185
stomat/o, 81
strept/o, 44
sub, 153
super, 144

Additional Word Parts

Following are some word parts that you can use with your word-building system. (There are others, of course, but these build fairly important and useful words.) If you want to enlarge your vocabulary dramatically,

1. choose a word part that interests you,
2. look for it in your dictionary
3. note how many words begin with this part,
4. list five of them with their meanings.

You may also find other words that contain the word part you worked with; for example, therm/o/meter and hyper/therm/ia.

WORD PART	MEANING	EXAMPLE
actin/o	ray	actin/o/dermat/itis
aer/o	air	aer/o/phob/ia
all/o	other, different	all/o/plas/ia
amb/i	both	amb/i/dextr/ous
ambl/y	dim, dull	ambl/y/op/ia
andr/o	man, male	andr/o/path/y
anis/o	unequal	anis/o/cyt/osis
antr/o	cavity, antrum	antr/o/scop/y
atel/o	incomplete, inperfect	atel/o/gloss/ia
audi/o	hear, hearing	audi/o/meter
balan/o	glans (penis or clitoris)	balan/o/plast/y
bar/o	weight, heavy	hyp/o/bar/o/path/y
bil/i	bile	bil/i/ur/ia
bi/o	life	bi/o/log/y
cac/o	bad, diseased, abnormal	cac/o/rhin/ia
cari/o	decay	cari/o/gen/ic
cat/a	down, downward	cat/a/leps/y
celi/o	abdominal region	celi/o/my/algia
cervic/o	cervix, neck	cervic/o/vesic/al
chir/o	hand	chir/o/megal/y

chrom/o	color	chrom/o/blast
chron/o	time	chron/ic
clas/ia	breaking	arthr/o/clas/ia
cleis/is	closure, occlusion	colp/o/cleis/is
coll/o	glutinous, jellylike	coll/oid
copr/o	feces, excrement	copr/o/stas/is
cry/o	cold, freezing	cry/o/therap/y
dacry/o	tear	dacry/o/aden/algia
dips/o	thirst	pol/y/dips/ia
doch/o	duct	chol/e/doch/itis
dyn/o	pain	cephal/o/dyn/ia
epipl/o	omentum	epipl/o/pexy
episi/o	vulva	episi/otomy
erg/o	work	syn/erg/y
es/o	within, inward	es/o/phor/ia
eu	well, easy	eu/phor/ia
febr/i	fever	febr/ile
gli/o	glue, neuroglia	gli/oma
gnath/o	jaw	pro/gnath/ia
hist/o	tissue	hist/o/tome
hyal/o	glassy, transparent	hyal/o/muc/oid
ichthy/o	fish	ichthy/osis
idi/o	personal, one's own	idi/o/path/y
in/o	fiber, fibrous	in/o/cyst/oma
labi/o	lip	labi/o/myc/osis
lal/o	speech disorder	ech/o/lal/ia
lept/o	thin, light, slender	lept/o/mening/itis
man/ia	mental disorder	megal/o/man/ia
mel/o	limb	hem/i/mel/ia
met/a	after, change	met/a/stas/is
morph/o	form	morph/o/log/y
myc/o	fungus	dermat/o/myc/osis
myring/o	ear drum	myc/o/myring/itis
nev/o	birthmark, mole	nev/o/carcin/oma
nyct/o	night	nyct/o/phob/ia
ocul/o	eye	ocul/o/nas/al
odont/o	tooth	odont/o/blast
olig/o	few, little, scant	olig/o/phren/ia
onc/o	tumor, mass	onc/o/lys/is
opt/o, optic/o	vision	opt/o/meter, optic/ian
orth/o	correct, straight	orth/o/scop/ic
osm/o	odor, sense of smell	an/osm/ia
ox/y	sharp, acute, acid	ox/y/cephal/y
pach/y	thick	pach/y/blephar/osis

papill/o	nipple-like, papilla	pappil/o/retin/itis
penia	decrease, not enough	leuk/o/cyt/o/penia
perine/o	perineum	perine/orrhaphy
phac/o, phako	lens of the eye	phac/oid, phak/o/cele
phall/o	penis	phall/ic
phon/o	voice	phon/o/graph
phor/o	bears, carries	o/o/phor/ectomy
phot/o	light	phot/o/therap/y
phren/o	diaphragm, mind	schiz/o/phren/ia
phyt/o	plant	dermat/o/phyt/osis
pil/o	hair	pil/o/cyst/ic
plat/y	flat, broad	plat/y/cran/ia
plic/i	fold	plic/a
poli/o	gray	poli/o/myel/itis
prot/o	first	prot/o/plasm
pseud/o	false	pseud/o/esthesi/a
pteryg/o	wing	pteryg/oid
rach/i, rachi/a	spine	rachi/o/dynia
radicul/o	root	radicul/o/neur/itis
sarc/o	flesh	sarc/oma
schiz/a, schist/o, schis/o	split	schiz/o/phren/ia
scoli/o	curved, curvature	scoli/osis
scot/o	darkness	scot/oma
seb/o	sebum	seb/orrhea
sept/o, seps/o	reaction against bacteria	a/sept/ic
sial/o	saliva	sial/o/aden/itis
sit/o	food	sit/o/therap/y
somat/o	body	psych/o/somat/ic
somn/o (/i)	sleep	in/somn/ia
sphygm/o	pulse	sphygm/o/man/o/meter
spondyl/o	vertebra	spondyl/o/lys/is
sten/o	narrowness, construction	sten/osis
stere/o	solid, solid body	stere/o/gnos/is
steth/o	chest	steth/o/scop/e
sthen/o	strength	a/sthen/ia
stigmat/o	mark, point	a/stigmat/ism
tel/e	distant, far	tel/e/metr/y
terat/o	monster, wonder	terat/oma
tetr/a	four	tetr/a/log/y
thant/o	death	thant/oid
trich/o	hair	trich/o/genous
trop/o	turning	heter/o/trop/ia
varic/o	varicose vein	varic/o/cele

ven/o	vein, vena cava	ven/o/clys/is
xen/o	strange, foreign	xen/o/phob/ia
xer/o	dry	xer/o/derm/a

Now hear the words from an expert's mouth.

It's a 60-minute pronunciation tape to help you with your newly-learned medical terminology. *Word parts* at the beginning of each chapter and *word lists* at the end of each chapter are pronounced so that you can compare your own pronunciation with that of the taped expert quickly and easily. This will aid you in checking your progress chapter by chapter. Medical terminology can be difficult to pronounce, but with your QUICK MEDICAL TERMINOLOGY Self-Teaching Guide and Audio-Cassette, the problem is solved! Fill out the postpaid order card below and mail today!

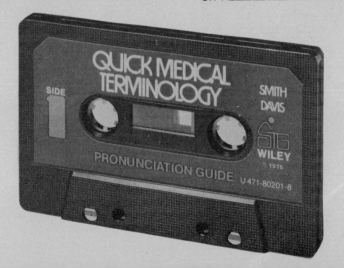

More Self-Teaching Guides to help you do your job better than ever!

QUICK LEGAL TERMINOLOGY
Randolph Z. Volkell, J.D.
You don't have to be a lawyer to understand one. All it takes is this simple guide to the main legal terms that often confuse laypersons. In the first half of this book, Volkell covers such topics as evidence, torts, contracts, business affiliations and commercial transactions, and wills, trusts, and family law. The second half features a glossary that acts as a convenient, permanent reference. Definitions include all the terms described in the first part plus many additional ones.
1979   (0 471 03786-9) $7.50

PUNCTUATION
Carl Markgraf, Ph.D.
Now there's an easy way for *everyone* to learn to use punctuation effectively in personal and business writing. Packed with examples, Markgraf's concise manual teaches this essential skill simply, by following common sense and using meaning and practicality as guidelines.
1979   (0 471 03100-3) $5.95

QUICK TYPING
Jeremy Grossman, Ph.D.
Touch typing for everyone who uses a typewriter or a computer keyboard—taught fast and painlessly by a tested and proven method. This practical guide gives you private touch typing lessons—at your own convenience. It also includes special backing sheets to make setting up forms, letters, and reports easy, and a mini style guide—a valuable permanent reference.
1980   0 471 05287-6 $6.95

QUICKHAND
Jeremy Grossman, Ph.D.
Teaches high-speed shorthand using just the letters of the alphabet and writing words as they sound. Instead of memorizing hundreds of special symbols, you learn brief forms of only 35 of the most frequently used words. A new, easy-to-learn, easy-to-use, practical shorthand based on scientific research and ideal for business, school, or personal use.
1976   0 471 32887-1 $5.95

HUMAN ANATOMY
Ruth Ashley
Teach yourself the basics of human anatomy and physiology—the structure, systems, and workings of the human body.
1976   0 471 03508-4 $7.95

Look for these and other popular Self-Teaching Guides at your favorite bookstore.
(Prices subject to change without notice.)

NO POSTAGE
NECESSARY
IF MAILED
IN THE
UNITED STATES

BUSINESS REPLY MAIL
FIRST CLASS   PERMIT NO. 2277   NEW YORK, N.Y.

POSTAGE WILL BE PAID BY ADDRESSEE

JOHN WILEY & SONS, Inc.
Attn: Quick Medical Terminology Audio Cassette
1 Wiley Drive
Somerset, N.J. 08873